BIOETHICS, GENETICS AND SPORT

Advances in genetics and related biotechnologies are having a profound effect on sport, raising important ethical questions about the limits and possibilities of the human body. Drawing on real case studies and grounded in rigorous scientific evidence, this book offers an ethical critique of current practices and explores the intersection of genetics, ethics and sport.

Written by two of the world's leading authorities on the ethics of biotechnology in sport, the book addresses the philosophical implications of the latest scientific developments and technological data. Distinguishing fact from popular myth and science fiction, it covers key topics such as the genetic basis of sport performance and the role of genetic testing in talent identification and development. Its ten chapters discuss current debates surrounding issues such as the shifting relationship between genetics, sports medicine and sports science, gene enhancement, gene transfer technology, doping and disability sport.

The first book to be published on this important subject in more than a decade, this is fascinating reading for anyone with an interest in the ethics of sport, bioethics or sport performance.

Silvia Camporesi is a Bioethicist with an interdisciplinary background in biotechnology, ethics and the philosophy of medicine. She is an Assistant Professor in the Department of Global Health and Social Medicine and Director of the MSc in Bioethics & Society at King's College London, UK. Over the past decade, Silvia has written extensively about the ethics of emerging biotechnologies. Her first book, *From Bench to Bedside to Track and Field: the Context of Enhancement and its Ethical Relevance*, was published for UC Medical Humanities Press in 2014. This is her second book. Silvia also serves as Associate Editor for the *Journal of Bioethical Inquiry*, and is a member of the Institute of Medical Ethics Research Committee, which fosters research and teaching in bioethics in the UK.

Mike McNamee is Professor of Applied Ethics and Director of the Research Institute for Ethics and Law at Swansea University, UK. Over the last 25 years he has pioneered the Ethics of Sport as a research field. He has published several books including *Research Ethics in Exercise, Health and Sport Sciences* (Routledge, 2006), *Sports, Virtues and Vices* (Routledge, 2008) and *Sport, Medicine, Ethics* (Routledge, 2016). He is the Founding Editor of the international journal *Sport, Ethics and Philosophy* (2007–17), and Co-Editor of Routledge's Ethics and Sport book series (1998–) which comprises more than 30 volumes. His work has been funded by various national research councils and the European Commission, in topics ranging from anti-doping policies and eating disorders in sport, to the ethics of human enhancement. He is a member of WADA's Ethics Panel, and Programme Director of a consortium of European Universities in a new Erasmus+ funded MA degree in Sport Ethics and Integrity.

ETHICS AND SPORT

Series editors
Mike McNamee
University of Wales Swansea
Jim Parry
Charles University, Prague

The Ethics and Sport series aims to encourage critical reflection on the practice of sport, and to stimulate professional evaluation and development. Each volume explores new work relating to philosophical ethics and the social and cultural study of ethical issues. Each is different in scope, appeal, focus and treatment but a balance is sought between local and international focus, perennial and contemporary issues, level of audience, teaching and research application, and variety of practical concerns.

For a complete series list please visit: https://www.routledge.com/Ethics-and-Sport/book-series/EANDS

Recent titles include:

Holism and the Cultivation of Excellence in Sports and Performative Endeavors
Skillful Striving
Edited by Jesús Ilundáin-Agurruza

Sport and Play in a Digital World
Edited by Ivo van Hilvoorde

Skills, Knowledge and Expertise in Sport
Edited by Gunnar Breivik

Doping in Elite Sports
Voices of French Sportspeople and Their Doctors, 1950–2010
Christophe Brissonneau and Jeffrey Montez de Oca

Bioethics, Genetics and Sport
Silvia Camporesi and Mike McNamee

Body Ecology and Emersive Leisure
Edited by Bernard Andrieu, Jim Parry, Alessandro Porrovecchio and Olivier Sirost

BIOETHICS, GENETICS AND SPORT

Silvia Camporesi and Mike McNamee

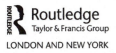
Routledge
Taylor & Francis Group

LONDON AND NEW YORK

First published 2018
by Routledge
2 Park Square, Milton Park, Abingdon, Oxon OX14 4RN

and by Routledge
711 Third Avenue, New York, NY 10017

Routledge is an imprint of the Taylor & Francis Group, an informa business

British Library Cataloguing in Publication Data
A catalogue record for this book is available from the British Library

Library of Congress Cataloging in Publication Data
A catalog record for this book has been requested

ISBN: 978-1-138-89223-1 (hbk)
ISBN: 978-1-138-89224-8 (pbk)
ISBN: 978-1-315-70925-3 (ebk)

Typeset in Bembo
by Taylor & Francis Books

Silvia: To future generations.
Mike: To Cher, with love.

CONTENTS

PREFACE

As every author will tell you, how a book looks when drafting a proposal for the publisher, and how it ends up, are often two different things. This particular book has been a long time in gestation. It is the product of a chance meeting at a Wellcome Trust funded symposium on bioethics and sport hosted at King's College London in 2011. Mike McNamee was invited by the organising team, which included Silvia Camporesi, and during the post-event dinner, the authors ended up chatting for hours on the intersections between ethics, sport and medicine. In the ensuing months and years we collaborated in several co-authored publications, many of which became the forerunners of the chapters that comprise this book. A full list of these essays is included in the acknowledgements. We are most grateful to the editors of these journals for their permission to reproduce parts of those essays, or a substantially modified version of those essays, in this book. Likewise we are grateful to the audiences of many national and international conferences in which the material was tested and refined.

We understand that many readers will come to the book without any knowledge of genetics. Others may approach the book with a great deal of knowledge of genetic science but no knowledge of ethics, medicine or sports, and so on throughout the various combinations of expertise or lack thereof among this triad. Attempting to accommodate the ranges of expertise and interest of the potential readership challenged us to present the material in ways that were both informative and interesting to novices but also engaging and provocative to experts. We have sought to cater for an audience that is, to some degree, informed in at least one of the three areas, which constitute the book's focus: bioethics, genetics and sports. In methodological terms, the book is a work of ethics that comprises both philosophical scholarship and relevant scientific and technological data, and the genetic and medical research therein. In ethical terms, therefore, the book is both one of descriptive ethics and prescriptive or normative ethics. We do not simply aim to describe or redescribe cutting-edge genetic research, all the latest arguments of bioethicists, or sports ethicists, but rather to undertake a critical review of these in order to arrive at normative judgements concerning existing and future policy and practice. What we have not attempted to do is to provide introductory overviews of the issues since these already exist in both bioethics and sport ethics literatures.

The book is self-consciously multidisciplinary in character, since the issues we address are of a kind not to be narrowly framed or solved. Bioethics is, by definition, multidisciplinary, and multidisciplinary scholarships always require a balancing act. We have attempted to reach out to a broad ranged audience that includes not just the bioethicists, genetic scientists, social scientists and sports ethicists, but policy scholars and practitioners too. To that inclusive end we include a glossary of technical terms in genetics in the appendix at the end of the book, but we assume a general ethical literacy and methodology.

The book is divided into two parts. Part I, *Genethics, Sports Medicine and Sports Science*, focuses upon genetic science research and technology in the contexts of Sports, Sports Medicine and Sports Science, and comprises Chapters 1 to 5. Part II is titled *Enhancement, Therapy, and the Ethical Construction of Categories in Sport* and encompasses Chapters 6 to 10.

In the first chapter we introduce the reader to key concepts in genetics and to the methodological approaches to the study of the genetic bases of sport performance. In line with the premise of the volume, which is to discuss realistic scenarios grounded in feasible science, and not to engage in science fiction thought-experiments, in Chapter 2 we focus on genetic testing for several conditions arising in sport such as (i) sudden-cardiac-death-related conditions; (ii) concussion-related trauma brain injuries; (iii) over-exertion complications related to sickle-cell anaemia trait; (iv) Achilles tendinopathies and anterior crucial ligament injuries. We show how these issues raise deep ethical questions concerning the paternalistic intervention of sports authorities over the lives of athletes, and the potential discriminatory consequences of their well-intentioned policies.

In Chapter 3 we look at one specific practice of genetic testing, aimed towards the identification of athletic talent. We point to the inherent problems of such testing, often driven by commercial products aimed at 'tiger' parents. We expose both the scientific shortcomings of such products through a philosophical analysis of the nature of athletic talent that forces a recognition of environmental influences on genetic predispositions. We also point out the perils of genetic determinism and the exploitation of public perceptions of the exceptional power of genetic data. A key element of our ethical appraisal is a fuller consideration of children's rights here and more generally the ethics of the child:parent relationship in order to avoid a zealous domination of the child by parental narratives.

How scientists gather and analyse data is the object of Chapter 4. Modern scientists are attempting to generate greater powers of genetic description and explanation of phenomena and this has driven a form of industrial mining of research data in what are called 'biobanks' or 'biorepositories'. The combinations of datasets allows for powerful analytical techniques to predict and control genetically linked conditions, but it also raises some key epistemological issues, mainly of two types: related to a presumed 'objectivity' of the data, and related to the context in which the data arise. Biobanking research also raises challenges to traditional forms of consent, the ethical authorisation that is essential to good biomedical research. Hence new models of informed consent have been developed for biobanking research that try to meet the unique epistemological challenges of such research. We present several such models, arguing for their benefits and weaknesses in ethical terms, and we apply this analysis to a new international biobank for sports genetics, the Athlome Consortium.

In Chapter 5, we analyse some feasible targets of gene transfer technology aimed at enhancing athletic performance, and engage with the ethical debate about whether genetic technologies aimed at enhancing performance are to be considered as a form of innovation or a new form of doping. There has been a tendency in some scholarship in bioethics and sports ethics to conclude that, because such rapid advances are being made, either we cannot predict the future or the future will be upon us swiftly and will be radically altered in the light of genetic advances. Many of the claims of the 2000s regarding gene doping, however, appear to have been hyperbolic. Humans are complex beyond genetic complexity, and sports are a wonderful combination of genotypical and phenotypical characteristics. In part, the chapter is a plea for more conservative estimations of the influence of genetic and medical science in sport thanks to a revision of our understanding of the limits of genetics.

In many ways Chapter 6 is the hinge of the book. While Part I has a greater focus on genetic research and technology in medicine and sports medicine, Part II of the book is more specifically applied to discussion of enhancement, identity and constructions of categories in sport. A large body of literature on the therapy/ enhancement distinction has arisen in the context of the goals of medicine. We survey this literature, and the more specific literature applying these concepts to the proper nature and goals of sports medicine. We present the thorny problems associated with the practice of seeking approval to use a therapeutic product that is also on the world anti-doping agency's list of prohibited substances and methods, for athletes who have a genuine medical condition that merits it. In discussing the pathological condition hypogonadism, we interrogate the case of athletes who gain approval for the use of testosterone, which would normally be thought of as a powerful hormone and illicit doping substance. By contrast we also discuss the possibility of an athlete who has a serious cardiac problem that requires treatment with beta-blockers, but who has been denied the use of such medication while competing in Paralympic sports events.

Pursuing the utility of, and problems raised in, the therapy/enhancement distinction, in Chapter 7 we discuss how a real-world gene transfer clinical trial of vascular endothelial growth factor has an ergogenic property that can work as a powerful therapy for pain control in a patient population, but equally as a powerful doping product in an athlete population. We employ here a comparative strategy to highlight the similarities and dissimilarities between the ethical frameworks used to evaluate the two scenarios. We argue that the context of gene transfer matters for the evaluation of the ethical desirability or permissibility of the experimental practice we are analysing: whereas the gene transfer trial to raise tolerance to pain may be ethically justified in a therapeutic context, the levelling out of pain from an endurance event undermines an essential component of the sporting contest, and the same gene transfer trial should be thought of as a doping product and thus prohibited in sports contexts.

In Chapters 8 to 10 we attempt to work through genetic and other medical ethical issues in the contexts of three athletic populations. Bioethical discussions have not always focused on the individual *within* classes or populations. We discuss the contentious problem of hyperandrogenism in athletics through the cases of Caster Semenya and Dutee Chand in Chapter 8. We lay out the regrettable history of gender verification testing in sports, and critically discuss its most recent pharmacological 'remedy' to the problem. We argue that forcing hyperandrogenic athletes to undergo testosterone depletion, as the IAAF and IOC would like to do, is ethically unjustifiable despite its purported justification to provide fairer competition among female contestants. We also recognise that it is not always possible to modify competition structures to accommodate fairness in competition, and in these cases we support inclusiveness, hence the inclusion of hyperandrogenic athletes in the female categories.

In Chapter 9 we set out the case of distinguishing congenitally impaired athletes from those who have acquired their impairments through a variety of life circumstances. We discuss the practical and ethical challenges of classification of Paralympic athletes but also we compare and contrast the cases of Oscar Pistorius and Markus Rehm as two exemplary contemporary cases of congenital and acquired disabilities respectively. We argue that while both have arrived at their impairments through different routes, each sport (running and jumping) has demands that compensatory or assistive technology may support or undermine. While this can be unproblematic in conceptual and ethical terms within classes of Paralympic sport, it can be problematic in sprinting and in long jump, especially, where the take-off phase may be radically enhanced by technological assistance.

Recent discussion of the genetic basis of sports performance have exacerbated racial discourse, although many of the racial assumptions remain problematically covertly hidden. In Chapter 10 we address the re-inscription of the concept of 'race' through sports in society and argue that it should have no place in sports genomics, nor in society. We also note how in some genetic scientific policies and practices the concept is sadly alive and well, and how in some recent sport journalism the concept of racial athletic superiority is being revivified in genetic clothing. We first explain how the use of the concept of 'human race' has no valid base at an ontological or epistemic level. We then proceed to spell out the ethical implications of the continued use of the concept of race in sport. We argue that this attempt to support the inferiority/superiority in modern sport and sports medicine in science through a re-inscription of the concept of race in genomics should be consigned to the dustbin of history. We conclude that the concept should be dropped altogether from genetic research, including in the context of sports and sports genetic discussions.

Our hope is that the book may break new ground by seriously juxtaposing the medical and sportive uses and misuses of genetic and other forms of biotechnology. It is clear that the logic of sports, to overcome invented difficulties in ways that do not offend formal and informal rule structures, is challenged every day by medical and scientific advances. Preserving the integrity of sport, while a problem for administrators, lawyers and politicians, is undeniably now a medico-scientific one too. We hope to have mapped some of the major contours of the genetic and bioethical threats to sport integrity here, and have attempted reasonably to propose ethically justifiable responses.

ACKNOWLEDGEMENTS

Silvia and Mike wish to express their gratitude to a plethora of conferences and audiences at which various incarnations of the book were presented and critically discussed, and from which we learnt much that contributed to the final volume.

A number of early versions of some of the material has been published in a variety of sport, medicine and bioethical journals and books, and we record our thanks to the various editors and publishers in the notes at the end of each chapter.

Several people have given feedback or helpful suggestions on specific portions of this volume. In alphabetical order, we would like to thank: Guido Barbujani, Andrew Bloodworth, Giulia Cavaliere, John William Devine, Brian Dolan, Steve Edwards, Javier Lopez Frias, Vanessa Heggie, Hiroaki Hobara, Søren Holm, Rod Jaques, Sigmund Loland, Sandy Montañola, Paolo Maugeri, Aurelie Olivesi, Jim Parry, Matt Perry, Wolfgang Potthast, Yannis Pitsiladis, Barbara Prainsack, Olivier Rabin, Markus Rehm, Sean Tweedy, Yves van Landewijck, Peter van der Vliet and Alan Vernec.

Silvia and Mike also wish to acknowledge the Wellcome Trust and King's Interdisciplinary Discussion Society for jointly funding the symposium in November 2011 at King's College London titled *Enhancement, Identity and Construction of Categories in the Olympics,* co-organised by Silvia Camporesi, Andrew Papanikitas and John Owens, where Silvia's and Mike's academic paths first crossed. Mike is grateful to the Wellcome Trust for sponsoring the *Genetics, Ethics and Sports Medicine* workshop at the International Convention on Science, Education and Medicine in Sport in Glasgow in 2012.

This book was finalised in the summer of 2017, when Silvia and Mike were able to get some time away from their teaching duties to complete the project. In particular, Mike expresses his thanks to Professor Ted Toadvine, Director of the Rock Ethics Institute, and Professor Nancy Williams, Head of the Department of Kinesiology, at Pennsylvania State University, for hosting him in the summer of 2017 which allowed much needed time, space and support for the finalising of the manuscript.

Both authors are grateful to John D. Davies for his meticulous proofreading of the manuscript. His work often went beyond mere proofreading by pointing out substantive comments that contributed to substantial improvements in this volume.

Silvia extends her gratitude to her husband, James Knuckles, and her extended Italian-American family, for being the best fan club possible. Mike, as ever, thanks Cheryl, Megan and Ffion for their forbearance and enduring love.

Finally, Silvia and Mike wish to express their deepest gratitude to Simon Whitmore and Cecily Davey at Routledge for their unwavering support and their patience with the gestation of this book.

Text acknowledgements

Chapter 2

Sections 2.2–2.5 draw upon material was previously published in a different version in Camporesi, S. and McNamee, M.J. 2013. Is there a role for genetic testing in sports? *Encyclopedia of Life Sciences Wiley Online Library*, Chichester, UK: John Wiley & Sons, Ltd. We acknowledge Wiley for granting us permission to reprint.

Chapter 3

The authors have been working on the topic of genetic testing for talent identification and development for several years, and have published several articles (co-authored, or single-authored) in this area. The articles are listed below. This chapter is substantially different from any of them, although naturally some of the ideas were developed for previous papers.

McNamee, M.J., Müller, A., van Hilvoorde, I. and Holm, S. 2009. Genetic testing and sports medicine ethics. *Sports Medicine, 39(5)*: 339–344.

Camporesi, S. 2013. Bend it like Beckham! The ethics of genetically testing children for athletic potential. *Sport, Ethics and Philosophy*, *7(2)*: 175–185.

Webborn, N., Williams, A., McNamee, M., Bouchard, C., Pitsiladis, Y., Ahmetov, I., Ashley, E., Byrne, N., Camporesi, S., Collins, M. and Dijkstra, P. 2015. Direct-to-consumer genetic testing for predicting sports performance and talent identification: consensus statement. *British Journal of Sports Medicine, 49(23)*: 1486–1491.

Camporesi, S. and McNamee, M.J. 2016. Ethics, genetic testing, and athletic talent: children's best interests, and the right to an open (athletic) future. *Physiological Genomics, 48(3)*: 191–195.

Chapter 4

A version of Sections 4.5–4.7 of this chapter was previously published as Consent, ethics and genetic biobanks: the case of the Athlome project, *BMC Genomics* (2017, 18(Suppl 8):830 https://doi.org/10.1186/s12864-017-4189-1), co-authored by Rachel Thompson and Mike McNamee.

Chapter 5

Some of the material included in this chapter was previously published in: Camporesi, S. 2014. *From Bench to Bedside, to Track & Field: The Context of Enhancement and Its Ethical Relevance*. San Francisco, CA: University of California Medical Humanities Press. ISBN: 978-0-9889865-4-1 (pp. 67–80). We would like to acknowledge Professor Brian Dolan, editor of UC Medical Humanities Press, for granting us permission to use the content in this volume.

Chapter 6

A portion of Section 6.2 was previously published in Camporesi, S. 2014. *From Bench to Bedside, to Track & Field: The Context of Enhancement and Its Ethical Relevance*. San Francisco, CA: University of California Medical Humanities Press. ISBN: 978-0-9889865-4-1. We would like to acknowledge Professor Brian Dolan, editor of UC Medical Humanities Press, for granting us permission to use the content in this volume.

Chapter 7

This first appeared in a shorter form in *Life Sciences, Society and Policy Journal* (2012), 8(1): 20–31 with the title Gene transfer for pain: a tool to cope with the intractable, or an unethical endurance-enhancing technology?, co-authored by Silvia Camporesi and Mike McNamee. The chapter has been substantially updated and extended for this volume.

Chapter 8

Parts of Sections 8.3–8.5 in Chapter 8 were previously published in a substantively different version in Camporesi, S. and Maugeri, P. 2016. Unfair advantage and the myth of the level playing field in IAAF and IOC policies on hyperandrogenism: when is it fair to be a woman? In S. Montañola & A. Olivesi (Eds), *Gender Testing in Sport: Ethics, Cases and Controversies* (pp. 46–59). New York: Routledge. We would like to acknowledge Routledge, an imprint of Taylor & Francis Group, for kindly granting permission to use the content in this volume.

PART I

Genethics, Sports Medicine and Sports Science

1

THE NATURE OF GENETICS AND ITS PLACE IN MEDICINE AND SPORT

1.1 Introduction

The aim of this chapter is to introduce the reader to key concepts in genetics and to the methodological approaches in the study of the genetic bases of sport performance. Genetic science and technology plays a key role in sport medicine and, hype notwithstanding, genomic science has made significant strides towards understanding the genetic pathways to sport excellence.

Casual use of the word 'genetics' can be confusing since it can be used in a variety of contexts, notably (i) genetic testing to test the predisposition to injury and response to training; (ii) whole genome sequencing of athletes to understand the genetic basis of sport performance; (iii) genetic testing to predict potential (talent identification and development); (iv) genetic technologies to enhance athletic performance. In each of these contexts, the use of genetics raises a plethora of ethical and epistemic issues, which we will discuss in turn in the following chapters. It may be helpful, however, if before exploring these complex issues we introduce some key terms that are integral to the debates concerning the use of genetics in sports.

Everything starts from our DNA. DNA stands for deoxyribonucleic acid. The iconic double-helix structure was unravelled by James Watson, Francis Crick, Maurice Wilkinson and Rosalind Franklin, at King's College London in 1951.[1] It is formed by four different nitrogen bases (adenine (A), thymine (T), cytosine (C) and guanine (G)) that bind in sequence and make a single DNA strand. Each base binds to its complementary base (A to T and C to G) to form a double stranded DNA. During replication the two strands open up and one copies itself to form another complementary strand that contains the same amount of genetic information. In these two strands all the genetic information – the blueprint of the information to codify for a member of a certain species – is included. Each triplet of bases codifies for an amino acid, one of the building blocks of proteins.

Genetics is a matter of genes, of course. However, what is a gene is not such an easy question; on the contrary, it is a philosophical question (Fox Keller 2000; Morange 2001; Nowotny et al. 2011)! One of the most important findings of molecular genetics is that the idea of a gene as a simple causal agent is not valid. The sequence of DNA that is referred to as a 'gene' has meaning only within a specific context, which determines its expression and function. That is why a single gene may have different effects depending on the context in which it is located (cellular context, environmental context, individual context, etc.). The human genome has about 21,000 genes and over 3 billion nitrogen base pairs, but note that of these 3 billion base pairs, only 5% are encoding regions, i.e. codify for proteins (Krebs et al. 2014). The remaining 95% used to be called until the early 2000s 'junk DNA', but it is now recognised that the term was a misnomer and is known that it plays a fundamental physiological role, especially in regulating the rate of gene expression. It is estimated that only 0.1% of the genome varies between individuals of the human species (see Chapter 10 for a discussion). For the purposes of this book, a gene is usually considered to be a specific region of the genome whose DNA sequence encodes for a discrete biological entity, usually a protein, but as we will repeat often throughout this volume, genes are not the only means of inheritance in the human species. As Jablonka and Lamb (2014) have identified, there are at least three other levels that determine the inheritance of traits: the epigenetic level (methylation and other modifications on the DNA that affect its function and expression and are passed down to future generations); and the behavioural and symbolic inheritance system, which together form what we usually refer to as 'culture'. Although we cannot enter into the philosophy of biology discussion of the different modes of inheritance in H. Sapiens, this volume is based on a strong premise that rejects any type of genetic determinism and exceptionalism.

By 'genome', we refer to the entire genetic material that is transmitted to the next generation. In the human species, it is for the most part encoded in the DNA sequence contained in the nucleus, although we have a small number of genes in the mitochondria organelles, which if mutated are responsible for some types of neurodegenerative diseases (hence, the mitochondrial replacement therapies approved by the UK Parliament in February 2015: Wolf et al. 2015).

Chromosomes are nothing other than discrete, compact units of the genome where DNA molecules are organised and that carry many genes. The human species has 23 pairs of chromosomes (each chromosome of the same pair is called homologous), which become unpacked during cellular division. There are two main types of cellular division: meiosis, the cellular division which takes place during sexual reproduction, and mitosis, the normal type of cellular division. With the word 'karyotype' we refer to the entire chromosomal complement of a cell or species, in the case of the human species, 23 pairs, XX for women, XY for men. A karyotypic analysis is typically performed during prenatal screening to establish the absence of chromosomal disorders, of which the most common is trisomy 21 or Down Syndrome (in which there are three rather than two copies of chromosome 21).

Each gene can occur in several possible forms, known as 'alleles'. In human beings, there typically are two alleles for each gene, one of which is located on each chromosome and one of which is inherited from each parent. For each gene, an individual can be homozygous, meaning having two identical alleles (either of the most common variant copy of the gene, or of the less common copy of the gene), or heterozygous, meaning having one allele of the most common copy and the other of the less common copy of the gene. Individuals are said to be hetero-zygous when they have different alleles at a particular locus, and homozygous when they have the same allele at corresponding loci on the homologous chromosome.

Traits that are controlled by a single gene are said to be 'monogenic'. In genetics, monogenetic traits are a minority, and result from modifications in a single gene. Common monogenic diseases are cystic fibrosis, thalassaemia, sickle-cell anaemia, Tay-Sachs, fragile X syndrome and Huntington's diseases. Monogenic diseases, although rare, affect millions of people worldwide. They are divided in three categories: dominant (a trait that needs to have only one mutated copy of DNA to appear phenotypically), recessive (a trait that needs to have two mutated copies of the gene to appear phenotypically) or X-linked (meaning that the gene causing the trait or the disorder is located on the X chromosome, leading to male/female differences in expressions, as females carrying two copies of the gene usually are healthy carriers of the disorder but do not normally express the symptoms, e.g. Duchenne muscular dystrophy).

'Haplotype' is a term that is used to refer to the particular combination of alleles in a defined region of a chromosome, while 'linkage' refers to the (probabilistic) tendency of genes to be inherited together as a result of their location on the same chromosome; it is measured by the percentage recombination between loci (see whole genome linkage studies below).

Penetrance refers to the extent to which a genetic variant has an effect on indi-viduals who carry it. In practice it is measured as the proportion of individuals that carry the mutated copy of the gene and express the phenotype (it is an indication of the 'strength' of the expression of the gene).

We refer to heritability as 'the proportion of the phenotypic variation in a trait of interest, measured in a given studied population and in a given environment, that is statistically co-varying with genetic differences (however measured) among individuals in the same population' (Kaplan 2015). Heritability is defined oper-ationally as the ratio of variation due to differences between genotypes to the total phenotypic variation for a character or trait in a population. It is a measure commonly used in twin studies in behavioural genetics.

Note that heritability is a technical notion which often gets misunderstood. One should never conclude from the mere fact that a trait is heritable that it is geneti-cally determined. Errors of reductionism and bio-determinism occur in statements such as 'Intelligence is 60% genetic and 40% environmental', or 'scientists have found that athletic excellence is x% genetic and y% environmental' and so on and so forth (see Chapter 10 for a discussion). 'Heritability is not a measure of "how genetic" a trait is. For heritability to make any sense at all as a statistic, the trait in question must vary in the population in question' (Kaplan 2015). It is important to distinguish familiality from heritability. Traits are familial if members of the same family share them, for whatever reason. Traits are heritable only if the similarity arises from shared genotypes.[2]

The term genotype refers to the genetic constitution of an organism, and is commonly found in opposition to phenotype, which refers instead to the appearance of an organism, resulting from the interactions of its genetic constitutions with the environment. We will often refer to genotype/phenotype interactions over the course of this book.

Another important concept in genetics, one that we will encounter often in this book in our discussion of the genetic basis of sport performance, is that of single nucleotide polymorphism (SNP), by which we refer to variations at the level of a single base pair in the DNA. These can be changes in a single base pair, deletions or insertions. When a variant appears in less than 1% of the population, it is generally considered a mutation (usually, with some health impact); when it is greater than 1%, it is generally considered a SNP. If the variations affect more than one base pair they are called polymorphisms, not SNPs. In that case there is a higher chance that there will be some effect on the phenotype.

1.2 Approaches to investigating the genetic bases of sport performance

Many, though not all, factors that are relevant for sport performance can be measured and quantified, such as body composition, aerobic power and muscle strength. Not all sports, however, are amenable to comprehensive quantitative measures of sport performance. Popular sports such as running, swimming and cycling are quantified by way of distance times. For many other sports, such as volleyball, tennis, rugby, football/soccer and gymnastics, among others, performance is not simply measured quantitatively; rather excellence is measured from a qualitative standpoint. John William Devine has developed a conceptualisation of the relevant types of sporting excellence in sport and how doping can be a threat to such relevant excellences (Devine 2010). This is only one reason why genotype–phenotype relationships are difficult to establish, and is something that must always be borne in mind when considering the results of association studies between traits that are alleged to be critical for success in this or that sport (Guilherme et al. 2014).

Although research into the genetic basis of sport performance has blossomed only in the last 15 years,[3] early studies date back to the end of the 1960s and the first research concerning the applications of genetics in sport. Those early studies concerned mostly the *phenotypic* characteristics of athletes, were focused on structural traits and were based on the statistical analysis of a given phenotype in the population studied. An example was the work carried out in 1968 during the Olympics in Mexico (De Garay et al. 1974). The purpose of the De Garay study was to test whether there was any association between participation in the Olympic Games and allelic variation in single-gene blood systems (Sawczuk et al. 2011, 254). The phenotypic variability they determined was the basis for studying the influence of genes on individual characteristics of the human body (ibid., 252).

In the early 1970s and throughout the 1980s, several studies into the effects of genetics on athletic performance were conducted. The main approach was based on twin and family aggregation studies. Klissouras and colleagues performed the first study on twins (39 pairs of twins) aimed at elucidating the correlations between genetics and adaptation to maximal effort. Their study concluded that 'there appears to be a significant resemblance in functional adaptability as measured by maximal oxygen intake between identical twins, whereas there is a divergence between non-identical twins' (Klissouras et al. 1973, 272) and paved the way for a spate of studies aimed at estimating the percentage contribution of genetic factors to common performance-relevant variables, such as bone density, muscle fibre type distribution, anaerobic capacities and so on. This enabled the identification of the levels of *heritability* of different complex traits. One of the most important projects of the last 25 years aimed at elucidating the role of genes in sport is the HERITAGE family study (the acronym derives from 'health, risk factors, exercise training and genetics'), commenced in 1992 and carried out until 2004 (Bouchard et al. 2000). The HERITAGE study demonstrated a variable degree of heritability for the different measurable aspects of sport performance, between 31% and 78%. Nevertheless, these early studies did not provide information about particular genes. The first polymorphism (ACE gene, more below) was identified only in 1998. Since then more than 200 SNPs have been identified; however, only about 20 have been replicated in subsequent studies and only one (alpha actinin gene) has been demonstrated to have a functional counterpart through animal studies (Pitsiladis et al. 2013).

There are several caveats that need to be pointed out concerning these studies if we are to proceed to a proper evaluation of them for our ethical discussion. To start with, it is important to note that although more than 200 polymorphisms have been identified, only about 20 of them have been identified in athletes. Many studies have failed to replicate the results, and we still know very little concerning *how* genes interact with each other and with environmental factors (Guth and Roth, 2013). This caveat is true for genetic science more generally, and is not merely valid for the more specific field investigating the genetic basis of sport performance. Moreover, as noted above, there are many traits related to sport performance that cannot, or cannot easily, be quantified.

There are three main approaches to investigate the genetic basis of sport performance (Guilherme et al. 2014). The first approach relies on candidate genes association studies, where a candidate allele is correlated with a targeted performance-relevant trait. These studies work in the following way: first, a physiological rationale to investigate a particular gene as a 'candidate' in the genetic basis of sport performance is established, based on what is known about the function of the protein codified by the gene. Then an association study is carried out – of which there can be different types. The first type of association study, the simplest, compares the frequency of genotypes in a cohort of controls (non-athletes) versus athletes, or compares a given intervention (e.g. exercise training or diet) between genotype groups (in this case the association studies are called 'longitudinal studies'). If the association study determines a statistically relevant significance for the candidate gene (or, better, allele), that needs then to be confirmed in another study that looks at how that particular allele affects protein expression, and how this affects the phenotype. This first step to establish an association between a 'candidate gene' and elite athletic status is not sufficient to accept a polymorphism as valid, and often associations found in a study are not replicated in subsequent studies. This limitation is very important to bear in mind when assessing the claims made by direct-to-consumer genetic companies concerning 'sports genes', which are analysed in Chapters 2 and 3 in this volume.

The second type of association studies that investigate the genetic basis of sport performance is more recent and is called genome-wide studies. This approach has advantages over candidate-gene studies as it allows the investigation of whole genomes instead than single genes (the advances in next-generation genome sequencing, with the concurrent lowering of the cost of sequencing, have made this possible). There are two types of genome-wide studies. The first type of approach studies genetic markers across the entire genome and is referred to as 'genome-wide linkage studies' (GWLS). Genes that are located on the same chromosome, or in adjacent regions within the same chromosome, share *genetic linkage*, which means that they have a high probability of being transmitted together to future generations. The proximity of two loci on a chromosome is measured by the percentage recombination between them. GWLS require familial data, as the basic unit of observations is a pair of individuals (usually siblings), and allow the identification of chromosomal regions that contain genes affecting quantitative traits over generations. GWLS have enabled the identification of a variety of traits associated with diseases, for example they have enabled the identification of alleles involved in type 2 diabetes mellitus and in rheumatoid arthritis (Stranger et al. 2011), but they have not enabled yet the identification of genes involved in sport performance.

More recently, with the decrease in genome sequencing costs, GWLS have been substituted by genome-wide association studies (GWAS) that analyse between 100,000 and several millions of SNPs across the genome, without any predetermined hypothesis about potential mechanisms (Yan et al. 2016). GWAS work by examining the association of genetic variation with outcomes or phenotypes of interest by analysing millions of SNPs across the genome. GWAS, contrary to GWLS, do not need to have a hypothesis about a candidate locus to operate, but polymorphism selection is based on observational data only. This is considered to be one of the main advantages of these studies, which, being 'hypothesis-free', allow the identification of new and often unexpected gene variants, and are considered to be more 'robust'. The downside is that they are still more expensive (hence their limited use) in sport sciences, although we can predict that this is likely to change in the near future, such is the speed of advances in the field.

1.3 Limitations

To date, GWAS have been successful in identifying genetic variations related to multifactorial diseases such as diabetes, among others. There are, however, important limitations in this approach that often go unnoticed or are glossed over by those interested in asserting with certainty the biological bases of a champion. The first of these limitations is the small effect size of most of the identified genetic variants. The number of participants (the size of the study) is perhaps the most important limitation of genetic association studies, and this limitation is exacerbated in elite athletes cohorts. It is critical to note that sample size is directly related to the statistical power of the study, and a limited number of participants can undermine our confidence in the conclusions of the study. When investigating the genetic basis of sport performance, this is the main scientific hurdle at present, as there are very few genetic cohorts of world-class athletes large enough to allow results that will have statistical power (Pitsiladis et al. 2013).

To give an idea of what results mean in context, a genetic variant in the percentage of muscle fibres affects only 2% of the total muscle fibres in an athlete's body. Therefore, inferences about the athletic performance of an individual with such variation are significant only to a very limited extent. Tests for ACTN3, which is often referred to as the gene for speed, are widely used by the companies selling tests online to the consumer. Height is another familiar example illustrative of this phenomenon. Human height is a highly heritable trait. At least 180 genetic loci have been associated with adult height, yet taken together these 180 loci still explain only about 10% of the variation in height, leaving the remaining 90% to be explained through interactions with environment and leaving much of the heritability of complex traits missing in scientific explanations (Yang et al. 2010).

A further limitation of GWAS is that the identified genetic variants often fail to show predictive utility, as these tests only detect statistical links between sequence variations in a particular genetic polymorphism and a phenotype. A statistical link does not prove that the gene variant is somehow implicated in disease development, nor does it tell researchers anything about the function of the gene and how it may be involved in the condition. Put simply, a statistical association cannot necessarily be assumed to have any clinical utility (Bhardwaj et al. 2004). Further functional studies aimed at elucidating the underlying biological mechanism of the gene involved, or, better, of the protein coded by the gene, still need to be carried out to demonstrate clinical utility. To date, there are no published studies using a GWAS approach in a cohort of athletes. GWAS of elite athletic performance are ongoing, aimed at identifying new SNPs that confer susceptibility to sprint and endurance performance by the use of world-class athletes (Jamaican athletes) as participants (Pitsiladis et al. 2013).

There is also an additional conceptual problem pertaining to the utility of these studies that should not be discounted, i.e. the definition of elite athlete. While it is common to refer to those who participate in international-level competitions as 'elite', to those who participate in national level as 'sub-elite' and to those competing in state and regional level competitions as 'non-elite', this definition is not used universally in the literature. Different authors, and therefore different studies, employ slightly different classifications (Guilherme et al. 2014; Swann et al. 2015). Moreover, even wherever there is homogeneity at the level of definitions, there are widespread national disparities in what counts as elite or sub-elite. Take the case of baseball, which counts as a professional sport in US, Canada and Japan, but not in other countries. Similarly, judo is a highly developed sport in Brazil, but not in New Zealand, while the reverse would be true of rugby. Many other examples are possible. That is why results inferred across countries may be obfuscated by different classifications, and by how the cultural context affects these definitions.

To date, the only allele that has been consistently identified and replicated as being associated with elite performance is the ACTN3 R577X polymorphism: the gene codes for the alfa-actinin 3 protein (Yang et al. 2003). As mentioned above, after a candidate gene has been identified replication is absolutely necessary to demonstrate the robustness of the alleged association. In addition, biological studies (animal models) looking at the inactivation of a certain gene (they are then called knock-out [KO] animal models) or overexpression of another (knock-in [KI] animal studies) need to be performed after a candidate gene has been identified. Validation and functional studies have been carried out in the case of ACTN3 R577X polymorphism: ACTN3 KO mouse models have been developed (they mimic the ACTN3 577XX genotype, i.e. deletion that is found in humans as an allelic variation), and studies have been carried out comparing KO to wild type (WT) mice. Such studies have confirmed that KO mice have reduced muscle mass due to the conversion of fast muscle fibres to slow muscle fibres, leading to an impressive increase in endurance capacity: KO mice can run or swim 33 times further than their WT littermates (MacArthur et al. 2007; MacArthur et al. 2008). The phenotype of the KO mice provides an explanation for the reduced sprint performance and improved endurance performance in humans with the ACTN3 577XX genotype, i.e. the deletion of the gene. Yet, to reiterate, this is the only gene/protein for which we have such robust data on the association with the phenotype, and for which we have animal models that can explain the phenotype in humans.

The ACTN3 R577X polymorphism is to date (Yan et al. 2016) the only gene that shows a genotype and performance association across multiple cohorts of elite athletes. That means that companies aiming at identifying gene variants involved in sport performance can legitimately make robust claims of clinical validity based only on the ACTN3 polymorphism. To conclude, as pointed out by Webborn et al. (2015), although a number of gene variations have been found to be associated with elite performance, generally these variations have tiny effect sizes and are heavily prone to type I statistical error, i.e. false positives. Notwithstanding the claims of companies selling the tests online or athletes' testimonials to the contrary, 'Current genetic testing is of almost zero predictive capacity' (Pitsiladis et al. 2013, 5). In the future priority should be given to recruiting sufficiently large study cohorts – which is going to be a major challenge for elite athletes, given also the difficulties in establishing a uniform definition of what counts as an elite athlete across nations, and the epistemological difficulties in classifying human beings, which we discuss in Chapter 10.

Notes

All websites accessed October 2017.

1 www.chemheritage.org/historical-profile/james-watson-francis-crick-maurice-wilkins-and-rosalind-franklin
2 www.ncbi.nlm.nih.gov/books/NBK22001/
3 One key article is that published by Yang et al. (2003), identifying an association between the alpha-actinin 3 gene and human elite athletic performance (see Chapter 3 for a discussion).

References

All websites accessed October 2017.

Bhardwaj, S.S., F. Camacho, A. Derrow, A.B. Fleischer and S.R. Feldman. 2004. Statistical significance and clinical relevance: the importance of power in clinical trials in dermatology. *Archives of Dermatology*, 140(12): 1520–1523.
Bouchard, C., T. Rankinen, Y.C. Chagnon, T. Rice, L. Pérusse, J. Gagnon and J.H. Wilmore. 2000. Genomic scan for maximal oxygen uptake and its response to training in the HERITAGE Family Study. *Journal of Applied Physiology*, 88(2): 551–559.
De Garay, A.L., L. Levine and J.E.L. Carter. 1974. *Genetic and Anthropological Studies of Olympic Athletes*. New York: Academic Press.
Devine, J.W. 2010. Doping is a threat to sporting excellence. *British Journal of Sports Medicine*, 45(8): 637–639.
Fox Keller, E. 2000. *The Century of the Gene*. Cambridge, MA: Harvard University Press.
Guilherme, J.P.L.F., A.C.C. Tritto, K.N. North, A.H. Lancha, Jnr and G.G. Artioli. 2014. Genetics and sport performance: current challenges and directions to the future. *Revista Brasileira de Educação Física e Esporte*, 28(1): 177–193.
Guth, L.M. and S.M. Roth. 2013. Genetic influence on athletic performance. *Current Opinion in Pediatrics*, 25(6): 653–658.
Jablonka, E. and M.J. Lamb. 2014. *Evolution in Four Dimensions, Revised Edition: Genetic, Epigenetic, Behavioral, and Symbolic Variation in the History of Life*. Cambridge, MA and London, England: MIT Press.
Kaplan, J. 2015. Heritability: a handy guide to what it means, what it doesn't mean, and that giant meta-analysis of twin studies. *Scientia Salon*. Available at: https://scientiasalon.wordpress.com/2015/06/01/heritability-a-handy-guide-to-what-it-means-what-it-doesnt-mean-and-that-giant-meta-analysis-of-twin-studies/
Klissouras, V., F. Pirnay and J.-M. Petit. 1973. Adaptation to maximal effort: genetics and age. *Journal of Applied Physiology*, 35(2): 288–293.
Krebs, J.E., E.S. Goldstein and S.T. Kilpatrick, eds. 2014. *Lewin's Genes XI*. Burlington, MA: Jones and Bartlett Learning.
MacArthur, D.G., J.T. Seto, J.M. Raftery, K.G. Quinlan, G.A. Huttley, J.W. Hook … and E.C. Hardeman. 2007. Loss of ACTN3 gene function alters mouse muscle metabolism and shows evidence of positive selection in humans. *Nature Genetics*, 39(10): 1261–1265.

MacArthur, D.G., J.T. Seto, S. Chan, K.G. Quinlan, J.M. Raftery, N. Turner ... and G.J. Cooney. 2008. An Actn3 knockout mouse provides mechanistic insights into the association between α-actinin-3 deficiency and human athletic performance. *Human Molecular Genetics*, 17(8): 1076–1086.

Morange, M. 2001. *The Misunderstood Gene*. Cambridge, MA: Harvard University Press.

Nowotny, H., G. Testa and M. Cohen. 2011. *Naked Genes: Reinventing the Human in the Molecular Age*. Cambridge, MA: MIT Press.

Pitsiladis, Y., G. Wang, B. Wolfarth, R. Scott, N. Fuku, E. Mikami and A. Lucia. 2013. Genomics of elite sporting performance: what little we know and necessary advances. *British Journal of Sports Medicine*, 47(9): 123–149.

Sawczuk, M., A. Maciejewska, P. Cięszczyk and J. Eider. 2011. The role of genetic research in sport. *Science & Sports*, 26(5): 251–258.

Stranger, B.E., E.A. Stahl and T. Raj. 2011. Progress and promise of genome-wide association studies for human complex trait genetics. *Genetics*, 187(2): 367–383.

Swann, C., A. Moran and D. Piggott. 2015. Defining elite athletes: issues in the study of expert performance in sport psychology. *Psychology of Sport and Exercise*, 16: 3–14.

Webborn, N., A. Williams, M. McNamee, C. Bouchard, Y. Pitsiladis, I. Ahmetov and P. Dijkstra. 2015. Direct-to-consumer genetic testing for predicting sports performance and talent identification: consensus statement. *British Journal of Sports Medicine*, 49(23): 1486–1491.

Wolf, D.P., N. Mitalipov and S. Mitalipov. 2015. Mitochondrial replacement therapy in reproductive medicine. *Trends in Molecular Medicine*, 21(2): 68–76.

Yan, X., I. Papadimitriou, R. Lidor and N. Eynon. 2016. Nature versus nurture in determining athletic ability. *Medicine and Sport Science*, 61: 15–28.

Yang, J., B. Benyamin, B.P. McEvoy, S. Gordon, A.K. Henders, D.R. Nyholt and M.E. Goddard. 2010. Common SNPs explain a large proportion of the heritability for human height. *Nature Genetics*, 42(7): 565–569.

Yang, N., D.G. MacArthur, J.P. Gulbin, A.G. Hahn, A.H. Beggs, S. Easteal and K. North. 2003. ACTN3 genotype is associated with human elite athletic performance. *American Journal of Human Genetics*, 73(3): 627–631.

2

WHAT ROLE FOR GENETIC TESTING IN SPORT?

2.1 Introduction[1]

There is a growing trend in sports medicine and sports science, which can be seen not only in the world of elite sports but also in general public policy, to utilise genetic technologies to predict and attempt to control the processes of our bodies. One particular instance of that trend is the use of genetic testing. Compared to other kinds of data, the power of genetic data is assumed to be exceptional. Within bioethics literature this phenomenon is referred to as 'genetic exceptionalism' (Bains 2010). It will surprise no one with any inkling of the powerful drives for performance enhancement that it has been applied within sports with some vigour. Starting from one of the premises of our volume, which is to discuss scenarios grounded in feasible science and not in science fiction, in this chapter we discuss genetic tests for injury prevention in four cases: (i) sudden cardiac-death-related conditions; (ii) concussion-related trauma brain injuries; (iii) over-exertion complications related to the sickle-cell anaemia trait; (iv) Achilles tendinopathies and anterior crucial ligament injuries. Beyond the role of testing as a potential precursor to therapeutic intervention, we also discuss the role of genetic testing for (v) training optimisation. We argue that there is, indeed, a role for genetic testing in sport, but only after some relevant distinctions have been made with respect to its aims; and even then, that role is a limited one. We do not directly discuss the more contentious issue of genetic tests as predictive of athletic potential. The cluster of issues that this innovation raises, particularly with respect to talent identification and development, will be discussed independently in the following chapter, while the cluster of ethical issues related to the application of genetic technologies to enhance athletic performance will be discussed in Chapters 5, 6 and 7 in this volume.

2.2 Genetic testing for sudden cardiac-arrest-related heart conditions

Sports develop their own micro-worlds, where play is somehow at one and the same time connected to and disconnected from the everyday world. There are periods in the practice of sport that throw up issues that force people to sit up and take notice beyond the score. The increasing prevalence of sudden cardiac arrest (SCA) is one such rupture of the everyday rhythm of sports. Sports, especially sports at an elite or even sub-elite level, present us with an image of incredible human vitality. To see that sapped by a SCA event is an almost perverse shock. Yet in sports of the US National Collegiate Athletic Association between 2004 and 2008 there were 237 deaths, 80 of which were attributed to medical causes (Harmon et al. 2011). The authors of this study conclude that SCA 'was the leading cause of death in 45 (56%) of 80 medical cases, and represented 75% of sudden deaths during exertion' (ibid., 1594). To the extent that sports medicine has a preventative goal, it is worth taking time to understand the aetiology of this phenomenon and its genetic basis.

SCA is defined as an unexpected arrest of the heart with potentially fatal consequences occurring generally within less than one hour from symptom onset in a person with a previously unknown cardiac condition (Sovari et al. 2011). Unsurprisingly, deaths resulting from SCA in high-profile athletes, sometimes broadcast live, have made media headlines in recent years: e.g. Boston Celtics basketball star Reggie Lewis dying from SCA on the basketball court during a practice in 1993, marathoner Claire Square collapsing and dying less than one mile from the finish line at the London Marathon in 2013, Italian soccer player Piermario Morosini suffering a fatal cardiac arrest during a match in 2012 (Vinocur 2011; O'Connor 2012). These broadcast deaths have sparked a debate on whether there should be a compulsory screening of young athletes for electrocardiogram (ECG) abnormalities, to prevent those from happening.

Most cases of SCA are related to different kinds of cardiac arrhythmias (irregular heartbeat patterns), with hypertrophic cardiomyopathy (HCM), a pathological enlargement of the heart, being the most common cause of sudden cardiac death in young athletes. However, it is difficult to estimate the prevalence of SCD with any validity, in part because of the difficulty in diagnosing the condition. SCA does not refer to a single pathological condition, but to a combination of conditions that exhibit the same potential fatal outcome (Koo et al. 2011). The physiology of the trained (and thus enlarged) heart of an athlete is similar to, and is often indistinguishable from, its pathological counterpart (George et al. 1991). Prolonged endurance training and static or power training produce changes in the structure and function of the heart, often presenting challenges to an accurate clinical diagnosis of cardiac conditions that genuinely present a risk to individuals (Myerson et al. 2012). Our awareness of the pathological potential of the enlarged athletic heart dates back to the 1950s. Only more recently were the physiological adaptations of the trained heart considered as a consequence of intense athletic participation (Heggie

2011). According to a recent review, however, the rate of sudden cardiac deaths among young athletes does not exceed 2 affected athletes per 100,000 per year (Farioli et al. 2015).

The first chromosome locus for the familial form of HCM and subsequent mutations involving the MYH7 (beta-myosin heavy chain) were associated with the aetiology of the condition more than 20 years ago (Marian et al. 1995). Since then, hundreds of mutations in more than 30 genes encoding different proteins related to the cardiac muscle have been identified (Bos et al. 2009). HCM is not a rare disorder. It affects 1 in 500 people and is characterised by extreme heterogeneity, both at the genotype and phenotype level and at the clinical course level: symptoms range from null to dyspnea or angina pectoris refractory to pharmacological treatment, to sudden death as the first and only symptom (Maron 2002; Bos et al. 2009).

The effect of the media spotlight can easily distort perception of contentious problems. The line between justified intervention in the lives of ordinary citizens and overbearing state paternalism is a hotly contested one (Feinberg 1986). With respect to SCA, the Italian government pioneered mandatory pre-participation screening of athletes. It was implemented as long ago as 1982, with systematic pre-participation screening that includes personal and family history, a general and medical cardiovascular examination and a 12-lead ECG (Myerson et al. 2012). The cardiac screening programme was not aimed only at elite athletes but was rather a public health intervention. Its scope was all individuals practising a sport at competitive level, which in Italy means being registered to a club (since the organisation of sport is not linked formally to the educational system). Hence anybody practising any sport as part of a club, or being registered to a gym, is obliged to undergo this kind of screening.[2]

This kind of mandatory screening was justified on grounds of being a useful public health tool. Elsewhere, for example in Denmark (Holst et al. 2010), the adoption of cardiac screening has not been thought of as sufficiently valuable to justify paternalistic intervention. This may in part be due to issues of prevalence, as highlighted by the Danish study. Nevertheless the Italian policy is not exactly an outlier in sports medicine and public health policy. The European Society of Cardiology recommends mandatory ECG screening of all competitive athletes (Corrado et al. 2005). So too does the Sports Science and Medicine section of the International Olympic Committee (IOC). By contrast, up until 2013, the American Heart Association and the American College of Sport Medicine (ACSM) recommended only a physical examination and family history questionnaire as a first-line screening, with further examination (ECG) based on the results of those initial steps, taking into account the economic evaluations of the high cost per person of screenings, due to the uniqueness of the US healthcare system (Halkin et al. 2012). Since 2013, new ACSM recommendations emphasise identifying those at greatest risk and classifying people as low, moderate or high risk based on the presence of different risk factors, including genetic markers, other signs or symptoms and cardiovascular, pulmonary, renal or metabolic diseases (Thompson et al. 2013).

It is fair to say, on balance, that the value of ECG and genetic screening itself for conditions related to SCA is contentious, as SCA refers to a combination of conditions that exhibit the same potential fatal outcome (Koo et al. 2011). Therefore, while genetic and ECG screening could identify individuals at a higher risk for some SCA-linked condition, others will inevitably be left out. Moreover, the test cannot predict the risk of death for any particular individual. Hence it is not straightforward – we argue it is a matter of ethical deliberation – what ought to be done with the result of the test. As noted above, the best estimate of the rate of SCA in the USA gives a figure of two deaths per 100,000 athletes per year (Farioli et al. 2015). What follows from this? If an athlete has a SCA-linked condition, her chance of dying each year during her professional athletic career is between 0.3% and 1% while younger than 35 years, as pointed out by Anderson et al. (2012).

To mandatorily screen athletes is one, not inexpensive, solution. Another option is to gain further knowledge about risk or pathological conditions that will allow more precise understanding and therefore predictive power regarding SCA. Yet greater knowledge of the condition does not automatically yield normative or policy directing conclusion. The question of how to use this knowledge remains, to a certain extent, open: it does not automatically follow that a positive test should result in automatic exclusion. If we believe that paternalistic intervention is justified on the basis of predictive screening, then we must also accept that mandatory exclusion of all at-risk athletes on the basis of ECG or genetic screening will exclude many who would never go on to suffer a SCA. Setting aside for a moment the concerns for the predictive ability of the screening – and these are not minor ones – there is another important point to be noted: would exclusion represent a justifiable infringement on people's autonomy, or freedom?

In Western democracies, we (generally) cherish various freedoms, often enshrined in legal rights that create a space in which we may pursue our self-conceived interests and projects. We might think of this space as both a logical and a political one. In the former sense it opens up a realm of options for action, some of which are critical to one's life and one's sense of personal integrity (often referred to as 'ground projects' after Bernard Williams (1973)), where one is said to be leading one's own life. The label 'agent sovereignty' (Arneson 1999: 16) has been coined to capture this idea and it coheres with senses of freedom that are deeply enmeshed in liberal worldviews (Berlin 1969). The classic statement of liberal freedoms draws upon the work of the nineteenth-century English moral and political philosopher and reformer John Stuart Mill. It is noteworthy for our purposes that it is directly related to a discussion of harm and the forms of responses to it when chosen by an autonomous individual. It is widely referred to as the 'harm principle'.

In a passage famous in modern moral philosophy, Mill writes:

> The object of this Essay is to assert one very simple principle ... the sole end for which mankind are warranted, individually or collectively, in interfering with the liberty of action of any of their number, is self-protection. That the only purpose for which power can be rightfully exercised over any member of

a civilised community, against his will, is to prevent harm to others. His own good, either physical or moral, is not a sufficient warrant. He cannot rightfully be compelled to do or forbear because it will be better for him to do so, because it will make him happier, because, in the opinions of others, to do so would be wise, or even right. These are good reasons for remonstrating with him, or reasoning with him, or persuading him, or entreating him, but not for compelling him, or visiting him with any evil in case he do otherwise. To justify that, the conduct from which it is desired to deter him must be calculated to produce evil to someone else. The only part of the conduct of any one, for which he is amenable to society, is that which concerns others. In the part which merely concerns himself, his independence is, of right, absolute. Over himself, over his own body and mind, the individual is sovereign.

(Mill 1859 [1989], 13)

We can apply Mill's line of argument directly to the case of athletes screened for SCA. Let us assume they have a reasonable knowledge of the facts, and the risks of SCA such as they may be reliably predicted. Suppose that an athlete chooses to go ahead and participate in competitive sport in the light of a positive screening. Certainly, if we are advocates of Mill's principle, their exclusion from athletic activity seems to be ruled out *tout court*. It seems that a variety of reasoned persuasion is all that is permissible. Education, broadly conceived, represents the limit of justified action insofar as one accepts the Millian position. As Mill says, our justified limits are 'remonstrating with him, or reasoning with him, or persuading him, or entreating him, but not compelling him' (ibid.). Of course, if there are harms to others, then our interventions find a ready justification. But it is not immediately clear that harm to others is a significant concern arising from the risk of cardiac arrest to the individual. This is not to say that others' interests in the continued life of the individual might not be worsened by the demise of the at-risk individual; only that intervening in their autonomous choices may not be justified. Anderson et al. (2012) adopt precisely this kind of liberal position in relation to the value of a robust SCA screening programme for the purpose of risk-awareness of the athletes:

Doctors can also play an important role in educating and interpreting the risk for athletes found to have an SCA-linked condition, but they are not the arbiters in deciding what level of personal risk is acceptable for an individual. Doctors can advise, but the final decision is not rightfully within their domain.

(Anderson et al. 2012, 332)

Along similar lines, Julian Savulescu, has also criticised the value of mandatory screening on the basis of its unwarranted paternalism (Savulescu 2005).

Mill offers a well-known caveat based on the notion of competence to autonomously decide a person's own life course. The presence of exceptions is of course well enshrined in law, and the use of surrogates to assist or sometimes replace those with immature or defective reasoning is relatively uncontentious. This autonomous capacity is widely referred to as 'competence'. One should note that particular persons are not, however, intrinsically competent or incompetent (Culver and Gert, 1982). Competence is a function of the relation between one's autonomous capacity and the object of a particular decision, which may be more or less complex – and thus place greater or lesser burdens on the informedness condition of consent. Hence, the point about screening children or young adults for SCA and possibly excluding them from competitive participation still holds as a potential justification. Such an act is considered a piece of 'soft' paternalism (Feinberg 1986). While the principle is fairly clear, its application is less so. Are parents justified in excluding their children from participation? Up to what age? In the UK, medical law has enshrined the Gillick competence, named after a mother who in 1983 sought an injunction against the medical doctor who prescribed an oral contraceptive to her 14-year-old child.[3] The test employed by the doctor concerning reasonable informedness of the decision was held up by the Law Lords on a majority basis. The criteria by which such a decision might be reached by a clinician became known as the Gillick Competence Test and aimed at assessing whether a child (understood in legal terms as a child up to 16 years of age) would be mature enough (i.e. competent) to give consent to his or her medical treatment, without the need for parental/guardian permission. The test is often applied in cases of sexual health, but was also recently applied in cases where the child's life was put at risk due to holding some deep-held belief (for example a religious belief about the forbidden nature of blood transfusions), which prevented treatment.[4] Often in the literature the use of Fraser Guidelines (enshrined in a 'Fraser competency form') has been recommended to determine competence. Thus the assessment of children's competence to undertake activity before or after screening might be something that could be guided by the Gillick Competence Test. Yet it is not straightforwardly obvious that taking a contraceptive pill at 13 is equivalent to a similarly informed adolescent classified as 'high risk' for SCA undertaking intense athletic activity that might predispose them to an untimely end. As Wheeler (2006) notes, the Fraser Guidelines are still used as legal guidelines specific to adolescent determinations of competence with regard to contraception. It would seem that a comparison of potential consequences might tip the scales in favour of soft paternalistic intervention. A survey published in 2005 and sent to registered clinical geneticists in the US, Australia and UK represents the largest study to date documenting instances of occurrence of genetic testing in young people for non-medical reasons (Duncan et al. 2005). Interestingly, the survey found that the most common justification cited for respondents' (who were clinical geneticists) views on the guidelines regarding predictive testing in young people was that each case needed to be considered individually, without sticking to a 'rigid cut-off' (ibid., 394).

What of those adults who are at risk of SCA? Ought we to sanction a 'hard paternalism' (Feinberg 1986) against them? It is rare enough for the state to intervene in such a way, though the mandatory wearing of seatbelts in cars, or of helmets when motor cycling, present us with widespread exceptions. Clearly the risk to such an individual is of the most serious kind. Nevertheless, the mitigation or acceptance of such interventions remains contentious. One possibility for those susceptible to this arrhythmia is the use of an internal cardiac defibrillator (ICD). The professional football player Anthony van Loo is famous not merely for being a Belgian first division footballer but also for suffering a cardiac arrest during a game with FC Antwerp in 2014. In video footage of the game he is seen to fall down after cardiac arrest only to sit up seconds later, the defibrillator having kicked in. Certainly we may say that spectators (and subsequent viewers of the video) have been shocked but not harmed. This raises questions about how risk should be assessed, by whom, to what degree and with what kind(s) of regulation, if at all.[5]

To conclude, further research needs to be performed to elucidate more precisely the genetic risk factors in sudden cardiac-death-related conditions, and to distinguish between them, but even if at a later point in time more robust screening programmes were available, we would object to their use for mandatory exclusion of competent individuals in professional sports. In this, we concur with both Anderson and Savulescu, since their position does not present a direct harm to others nor to the social good of sport itself. Our acceptance of their liberal position does not extend to all ethical issues in sport since, as in the case of doping, there are other ethical notions that come into play, which we discuss in Chapters 5 to 7 in this volume.

2.3 Genetic testing for concussion-related traumatic brain injuries[6]

In the last few years a number of sports, including Australian rules football, rugby union, rugby league and most especially American football, have been at the centre of a strident public debate due to the recent wave of suicides in college footballers after concussion-related permanent trauma brain injury (TBI), also known as chronic traumatic encephalopathy (CTE) (Park 2010; O'Connor 2012). The controversy has even spawned a 2015 Hollywood blockbuster, titled *Concussion* (with tagline 'Tell the Truth') and featuring the well-known American actor Will Smith as a forensic pathologist fighting against the US National Football League trying to suppress his research on how repeated trauma on the field of play leads to CTE.

It may come as a surprise to some readers, though not to clinicians nor to philosophers, that the definition of concussion is contested (McNamee et al. 2015). An operational definition, not aiming at technical complexity, is that concussion is an event that occurs when the brain hits against the skull as a consequence of the application of force (Hecht 2002). It is thought that sport-related concussions (SRCs) are a precursor to CTE (Gavett et al. 2011). The definition of CTE is also under discussion (although less contested than concussion), it being a syndrome, i.e. a condition characterised by a set of different symptoms that can be caused by different causes. CTE is generally defined as a progressive degenerative disease of the brain that is found in individuals with a history of repetitive brain trauma, including but not restricted to concussions. The syndrome has long been recognised – since the beginning of the twentieth century – in professional boxing, where it was referred to as 'dementia pugilistica', because professional boxers were the first to be known to develop the syndrome following repeated blows to the head (Millspaugh 1937). As reported by McKee et al. (2009), the concept of CTE was first pointed out in 1928 by Martland, who introduced the term 'punch-drunk' to refer to a group of symptoms that seemed to be the result of repeated sub-lethal blows to the head. In CTE, repetitive trauma initiates progressive degeneration of the brain tissue. The abnormal form of the protein tau, also found in Alzheimer's-disease-affected individuals, accumulates in the brain of individuals with CTE. These anatomical pathological changes in the brain do not start taking place immediately upon the onset of SRC, but they occur typically years after the last brain trauma or the end of their athletic career. The degeneration of the brain is associated with a plethora of symptoms: from progressive memory loss, to impaired judgement, to impulse control problems often manifested as aggressive behaviour, to depression and finally to dementia (McKee et al. 2009). On top of these difficulties, there is no treatment and no definitive pre-mortem diagnosis, as the only definitive diagnosis is made at autopsy, when the distinct neuropathology consisting of deposition of perivascular hyperphosphorylated tau (ptau) protein is confirmed (Saulle and Greenwald 2012; Verscaj et al. 2017).

By the end of 2012, thousands of former professional football players had filed lawsuits against the NFL (the US National Football League) accusing the league of hiding information about the long-term harms derived from concussions on the field of play (Park 2010). The precise incidence of CTE after repetitive head injury is unknown, however, and it is thought by some to be much higher. It is also unclear what severity or recurrence of head injury is required to initiate CTE (McKee et al. 2009). This has led some philosophers to call for the elimination or prohibition of American football (Corlett 2014; Sailors 2015), though others are for the present more sanguine (Lopez Frias and McNamee 2017), based on a consideration of the facts as currently known.

In contrast to the neuroscientific viewpoint of McKee and others, a series of global consensus statements from a cohort of leading neuroscientists and clinicians, calling themselves the Concussion In Sport Group (CISG), have drawn more conservative conclusions about the relations between blows and jolts to the head and the onset of CTE (see for example McCrory et al. 2013). In their most recent systematic review, the CISG authors write that they screened 60,000 articles regarding SRC. In relation to CTE they report that:

> The potential for developing chronic traumatic encephalopathy (CTE) must be a consideration, as this condition appears to represent a distinct tauopathy with an unknown incidence in athletic populations. A cause-and-effect relationship has not yet been demonstrated between CTE and SRCs or exposure to contact sports. As such, the notion that repeated concussion or subconcussive impacts cause CTE remains unknown.
>
> *(McCrory et al. 2013, 7)*

The CISG have drawn some criticism for their close relations with professional sporting bodies (Partridge 2014; Partridge and Hall 2014). As we noted above, the terrain of SRC is contested at conceptual, scientific and clinical levels, albeit to differing degrees. How does this contentious issue relate to our present nexus of genetic concerns?

As in all diseases, genetic factors contribute to the development of CTE. In particular, the allele epsilon 4 of the apoliprotein E (APOEε4) has been robustly associated with Alzheimer's disease, and is now thought to play a role in the development of CTE. Although there is some evidence suggesting that APOEε4 confers risk for CTE, it is not known whether APOEε4 is a risk factor for the hyperphosphorylation of the tau protein (influencing the severity of the disease), or whether the effect is modified by repetitive head impacts (Verscaj et al. 2017).

Savulescu (2005) has advocated the benefits of voluntary testing to identify groups at increased risk in the boxing world. Nevertheless, consistent with his other writings, he adopts a strong liberal position according to which individuals should be left free to decide – whether in the context of sport, or in any other context of life – the type of risks they want to run. He writes: 'Vigorous promotion of understanding of risk is consistent … with the duty of beneficence and with the respect of individual autonomy' (ibid., 145). He also highlights how there might be indirect benefits not only for the individual being tested but for society at large, if boxers (in the context of screening for APOEε4) decide to opt out of, or cease, their participation. In doing so the state is relieved of the burden to pay for their healthcare in case of development of CTE. This is one specific aspect of Corlett's arguments. His argument is that the harms voluntarily incurred by American football players place an unjust burden on taxpayers, since the players will not be able to pay for their complex long-term care (Corlett 2014). For Corlett this amounts to a case for prohibition, whereas Savulescu stresses how the screening and the opt-out need to remain on a completely voluntary basis (and here there might be some tension with the indicated indirect benefits to society).

In an editorial for *Science & Translational Medicine*, Gandy and DeKosky raise the question of whether screening for APOEε4 allelic variant could help in identifying individuals at higher risk of developing CTE following concussions either on the field of play (for athletes), or on the battlefield (for military personnel) (Gandy and DeKosky 2012). Gandy and DeKosky also conducted a preliminary survey among experts in Alzheimer's disease TBI and CTE regarding the value of introducing APOE genotyping. The consensus resulting from the poll was clear: most of the interviewees agreed that it is premature to introduce APOE genotyping for several reasons including the lack of a systematic registry, screening or genotyping of at-risk individuals, and the fact that most existing data on APOEε4 and dementia risks are healthy controls in their mid- to late life, so these results cannot be extrapolated to athletes at risk for CTE whose exposure may begin during adolescence (ibid.).

Notwithstanding the data on the prematurity of genotyping for APOE, some companies are already offering testing for the APOE allele sold online 'directly to the consumer', claiming it can be useful in informing coaches and athletes alike about return-to-play decisions. Athleticode was a case in point. We could read the following claim on their website:

> Enough studies have been conducted to allow this information to be incorporated into the educational repertoire of physicians, athletes and their parents in developing a return to play plan of action after sport concussion. Athleticode's APOE test identifies several specific regions along the Apolipoprotein E gene … Athleticode's APOE test provides information that a physician, athletes and their parents can consider and use in deciding upon a return to play plan after TBI.[7]

It is our judgement that claims such as this one by Athleticode are seriously problematic: the problem of concussion and return-to-play decisions cannot be swept 'under the carpet' (i.e. summarily solved) with DTC-genetic tests. Rather, policy and practice changes must be confronted by rules changes and stricter implementation of sanctions on, for example, lawful head contact in rugby tackling, or helmeted collisions in American football. Moreover, the very design of helmets or headgear in equestrianism, boxing, ice hockey and American football should be seriously addressed with a range of other prevention strategies. This will not be easy. In contact sports such as American football, ice hockey or rugby, 'hard hits and head collisions are more than simple aspects of the game; they are part of the sports' identity', as Saulle (2012) notes, and are also a facet of marketing and media commodification.

The issues surrounding head injuries will be familiar to anyone who has followed the debates on the legalisation or outlawing of boxing. Among the myriad of ethical arguments, one key dimension is whether blows to the head might be removed from the range of permissible actions of boxing (Dixon 2001; Radford 1988). Now those who are paternalistically inclined will say that this simple rule change will bring about significant harm reduction. There are two counters to this by proponents of boxing: the first is an empirical claim, the latter – a more fundamental – conceptual one. If the head is removed as a legitimate target, knockouts are far less likely, and so it is feasible that boxers will receive even greater 'punishment', though simply to other organs or parts of the body. This may or may not be the case. There is no sufficiently reliable evidence base to work from yet; hence the need for more precise empirical data. The second claim is more fundamental and pertains to the nature of the activity: without the head shots, boxing would be a different activity altogether, which we could call – let us say – *boxing1* and not boxing per se. This argument may be sound but is not decisive in deliberating about what to do regarding head shots. What we are left then with is a question of whether we prefer one version of the activity to the other, and on what basis we make this decision. A similar rule change has been made in amateur boxing, after all, where the wearing of padded headgear is compulsory, and where there are shorter and fewer rounds in which to harm, or excel, or both.

In sports such as American football where helmet wearing is compulsory, further problems arise. When the rule change happened to make helmet wearing compulsory in 1943 (MacIntyre 2016), it seemed that the strategies of the game changed too. Helmets could be seen as both protective and as an offensive tool. Some have questioned, analogous to our boxing example above, whether this fact has played a role in the increase of head injuries. As noted by Goldberg (2009), 'No helmet can prevent the brain from striking the interior of the cranium upon the application of adequate force'. As with boxing, then, questions of harm come into focus alongside ethical questions of what we think of contests like those in ice hockey or American football. What ought to be understood as an intrinsic feature of the game, and what ought not, are philosophical questions. What kinds of harms arise with what kinds of certainty is both an empirical and a philosophical question, since not all injuries will be thought of as serious enough to merit the description 'harmful'. Some of these injuries and harm will be susceptible of genetic answers in part. Yet even when these are settled, there will of course be the key political question: who ought to decide?

At present helmet wearing is compulsory in ice hockey and American football, though protective headgear in rugby is a voluntary choice, as long as it conforms to certain standards (McIntosh and McCrory 2005). The uncertainty of the safety of return-to-play decisions after a concussion has slowly come to be recognised and disclosed to the player-patient. That is why prevention requires a complex approach involving all stakeholders, from coaches to players, to team doctors, to referees and the public (Saulle and Greenwald 2012). It is possible that only the threat of mass torts (as are ongoing in the USA from former NFL players) will drive rule and culture change.

As noted above, Savulescu (2005) has criticised the value of mandatory screening in the boxing context on the basis of its illiberality and infringement of one's autonomy. When, however, is it sufficient simply to point to the restriction of freedoms to harm oneself as one rationally chooses? Clearly in the case of American football, boxing, cycling, equestrian sports, ice hockey, formula motor racing and other sports with intrinsic risks to athletes' safety, individuals engage in practices that bring about complex combinations of pleasure and pain. Moreover, they do so in a public sphere where serious concerns are raised about other ethical issues concerning role modelling, the support for norms of more or less legitimated aggression or violence, and so on. A key series of issues arise in relation to the assumption and mitigation of risk to athletes' welfare. There will be occasions where the liberal autonomy-respecting viewpoint will be unproblematic, and there are exceptions within the liberal position for incompetent or vulnerable populations. It may also be the case that a more communitarian perspective, where supra-individual stakeholders (community groups, clubs, even the state) may seek to intervene in those freedoms, where the risk of developing or triggering potentially fatal conditions may be thought to present a serious threat or offence to ethical norms.

2.4 Genetic testing for complications related to the sickle-cell anaemia trait

In April 2010, the National Collegiate Athletic Association (NCAA), which supervises the athletic programmes at colleges and universities in the US and Canada, mandated genetic testing for sickle-cell anaemia, effective 1 August 2010, for all student athletes in Division I, the highest level of college athletics (Thomas and Zarda 2010). The mandatory testing was part of a settlement reached in response to a lawsuit brought forward by the family of Dale Lloyd II, a student at Rice University (Houston, Texas) who died aged 19 years old, after a particularly intense football practice in September 2006.[8] At autopsy his death was attributed to 'acute exertional rhabdomyolysis' (i.e., destruction of skeletal muscle fibres resulting in the release of myoglobin and other cellular contents in the circulation, with toxic effects on the kidneys and potential kidney failure), one of the rare consequences of sickle-cell anaemia trait, a trait that Dale Lloyd II carried (Tsaras et al. 2009).

Sickle-cell disease is a monogenic recessive genetic disorder caused by a single mutation in the β-globin gene. Its molecular aetiology was determined by Linus Pauling, who in 1949 named it a 'molecular disease' (the first of many to come) and who later was awarded the Nobel Prize for his discovery (Pauling et al. 1949). The sickle shape of the mutant cells is the basis of the pathophysiology of sickle-cell anaemia, which is characterised by chronic anaemia, haemolysis (rupturing of red blood cells with the release of their content into the plasma) and results in a range of symptoms, ranging in severity from fatigue; pain crises; different degrees of swelling and inflammation of joints; opportunistic bacterial infections; and in the most severe cases to liver congestion, lung and heart injury, which can be fatal. The vaso-occlusion (blockage of arteries) is also typical of the disease, and is caused by the obstruction of circulation by the sickle-shaped cells (which literally occlude the blood vases due to the shape of their cells). This blockage of the arteries in turn leads to ischaemic injuries and potentially fatal major ischaemic injuries during crisis, which can be triggered by over-exertions on the field of play, like the one that was fatal to Dale Lloyd II.

Individuals with only one mutated HbS gene are carriers of sickle-cell anaemia, and can be also referred to as having the 'sickle-cell trait'. That means that in normal everyday life conditions carriers of the trait do not experience symptoms. Under conditions of over-exertion – such as intense exercise, or in cases of lessened intensity but high temperature environments – they can experience complications (Tsaras et al. 2009). From an evolutionary standpoint, there has been a positive pressure to select for the HbS heterozygous individuals (the carriers of the disease, who are asymptomatic of most conditions except when they encounter areas of low oxygen pressure) because they exhibit a higher resistance to infection to *Falciparium malaria*, the parasite that causes malaria. This is because of the shape of their red blood cells which are less hospitable to the parasite (Rees et al. 2010). Due to the survival advantage conferred by the sickle-cell heterozygosis, the prevalence of the sickle-cell trait is higher across equatorial Africa (where malaria is endemic), ranging between 10 and 40% (Ashley-Koch et al. 2000) In the US, prevalence of the sickle-cell trait is approximately 8% in people of African descent and 0.05% in white Americans (Tsaras et al. 2009).

It must be noted that the NCAA mandatory genetic testing policy (a result of the settlement with Dale Lloyd II's family, as noted at the beginning of this section) applies to every student athlete in Division I. It does not mandate exclusion from professional athletic participation, but recommends changes in training – less intensity, better hydration and less exposure to heat – as these could be triggering factors for the sickle-cell-anaemia-related complications described above. It is important to note that while prevalence of sickle-cell anaemia can only be estimated, one recent study reported that over 2,000 NCAA Division I student-athletes with SCT will be identified under this screening policy (Tarini et al. 2012). This is why, notwithstanding the useful recommendation for changes in training, and not exclusion, the new NCAA policy has sparked controversy. Critics have been concerned that this may be a form of indirect discrimination against groups of carriers, since the prevalence of the sickle-cell trait is higher in African Americans as explained above (Stein 2010). How could such a well-motivated position be discriminatory in practice? The answer is that implicit exclusion policies result in unintended outcomes when training regimes cannot easily be altered in the exceptional conditions of elite and sub-elite sport.

Screening for sickle-cell anaemia might have prevented Lloyd's death by tailoring practice to his condition, if possible, for example, by avoiding some training conditions. The extent to which this would have been done with his cooperation or as a hard paternalistic intervention is a moot point. Moreover, one could argue that this is difficult to avoid in many competitive sports by virtue of the physical intensity intrinsic to the activities. Alternatively, a mandatory screening coupled with a strong paternalistic policy of exclusion (implicit or explicit) could have prevented him from participating in high-level collegiate sport in the first place.

In January 2012, the American Haematology Association (AHA) released a statement outlining its opposition to sickle-cell anaemia mandatory screening on the basis that:

> Screening alone is an extremely limited approach intended to protect the liability of the NCAA and the athlete's university, not the student athlete … Furthermore, sickle cell trait is not the only condition that can lead to death from athletic over-exertion, underscoring the need for the NCAA to require universal preventive interventions in its training programs that will better protect everyone.[9]

Our evaluation of mandatory screening for sickle-cell anaemia is twofold. First, we concur with the AHA opinion stating that the NCAA should implement universal, comprehensive programmes for the prevention of sudden-death-related conditions on the field of play, as the preventative measures spelled out above to avoid sickle-cell trait complications would also serve potentially as good preventative measures to avoid dangerous over-exertion-related injuries in all student athletes. We also recognise, however, the potential harm that could derive from discrimination or targeting of carriers, especially in relation to the higher prevalence in African Americans. Group discrimination is one of the possible risks related to biobanking research projects, as we discuss in Chapter 4 in this volume. Second, we recognise the benefits of genetic screening for the sickle-cell anaemia trait, particularly in that it can help identify individuals at a higher risks of over-exertion-related injuries and complications, and tailor *ad hoc* training programmes to specific athletes. We see this development as an important point of departure in discussions concerning the duties of colleges or universities to their student athletes, especially since these are highly commercialised entities where the key actors in the event are not justly remunerated (Pielke 2016; Morgan 2017). The AHA has explicitly acknowledged that 'the NCAA Division I policy has the potential to harm the student athlete and the larger community of individuals with sickle cell trait'.[10]

To the best of our knowledge, there are no other similar screening programmes implemented at the level of college or professional sport apart from the NCAA's mandatory genetic testing. It must also be noted that student athletes can avoid testing by signing a waiver releasing the NCCA from liability (although of course this would just shift the burden of the disease and its consequences on to the athletes themselves) (Bonham et al. 2010). While not a solution to all athletic sudden death scenarios, we think the screening programme is still meritorious, especially when combined with proper educational messages to players, coaches and athlete support personnel such as sports medicine professionals, or strength and conditioning coaches. At the moment, such additional measures are not part of NCAA policy, which is problematic (Abkowitz 2013). We conclude that the potential benefits of genetic screening for sickle-cell anaemia outweigh its downfalls. We therefore recommend that the NCAA should keep in place its mandatory screening for Division I athletes and consider expanding it to Divisions II and III athletes who also undergo intense training.

2.5 Genetic testing for Achilles tendinopathies and anterior crucial ligaments ruptures

While not as dramatic or as eye catching as life-threatening conditions such as sudden cardiac death, concussion or sickle-cell anaemia, Achilles tendon and anterior cruciate ligament (ACL) injuries are one of the most severe injuries sustained during participation in sport, with athletes potentially losing several months of play (September et al. 2012). In some populations, young and old, these may be career-ending (or, for amateurs, sport-terminating) injuries. These injuries are exceptionally common not only in sport, as a retrospective 10-year study conducted by Raikin and co-authors of more than 400 Achilles tendon ruptures occurring in the US from 1992 to 2002 demonstrates (Raikin et al. 2013). This study has identified that 68% of the total number of men and women diagnosed with Achilles tendon ruptures in the US are due to sport participation, with basketball being the most common cause, followed by tennis in second place and by football in third place.

Genetic factors are among the risk factors that have been implicated in the etiology of both conditions (Collins and Raleigh 2009). In particular, several polymorphisms located within the genes encoding for collagen chains (COL1A1, COL12A1) and matrix-metalloproteinases (MMP12) have been associated with both events (September et al. 2012) Moreover, it has been demonstrated that individuals who carry a particular single polymorphism in the gene encoding for GDF5 (growth-differentiation-factor 5, a protein member of the bone morphogenetic protein (BMP) family and the TGF-beta superfamily) have twice the risk of developing an ACL pathology compared with non-carriers (Posthumus et al. 2010). Several patents have already been filed on the basis of these results for genetic tests aimed at testing either independently or collectively these specific polymorphisms, and to see how they interact with each other or with other polymorphisms to modify the risk of either tendon or ligament injuries (September et al. 2012).

The ability to identify subgroups of individuals at higher risk of developing tendinopathies through genetic tests is very valuable to professional sports franchises as well as individual athletes (Scott et al. 2011). It is important to note that none of the identified genetic polymorphisms independently cause Achilles tendinopathy or ACL injuries, merely that they are significantly correlated with such injuries. That is to say, that certain polymorphisms modulate or contribute to the risk for these injuries. Therefore, none of these genetic tests are diagnostic in nature, but they could be helpful in a programme of reducing the risk of injury in high-risk athletes by personalising their training programmes, rather in the same way that training might be tailored to sickle-cell anaemia athletes as a risk mitigation strategy. As noted by September and co-authors, it is vital that *all* risk factors (genetic and non-genetic) be incorporated into a multifactorial model to predict risk for Achilles tendinopathies and ACL ruptures. These injuries are not life threatening but, given their prevalence and significance for efficient human movement, the aim should be to increase athletic longevity, which would be a positive outcome not only for individuals but also for clubs and colleges.

Goodlin et al. argue similarly that genetic testing 'may aid in the development of tailored injury prevention program for athletes, which could provide a new edge for successful competition' (Goodlin et al. 2015, 2). Precisely who should pay for such a testing regime is a moot point. In professional sports, medical insurance policies might well consider such tests as important in pre-contract discovery and negotiation. The range of uses might both serve to undermine athlete interests or to secure them, depending on the results and on who has access to them. These tests have a high commercialisation potential. Professional football (soccer) teams in the English Premier League have already expressed an interest acquiring these tests for analysis, and apparently the English Institute of Sport (the UK's largest provider of sport science, medicine and technology, offering consultancy to coaches and trainers 'to improve the performance of their athletes') has expressed interest in acquiring genetic testing for Britain's Olympic athletes (ibid.).

What is clear, however, is that such information from genetic testing is only part of the story. A more general point here must be made, which applies to each of the potential genetic testing and screening cases instanced above. What do the data that are produced actually mean, how should they be interpreted and used to guide athletic and medical decision-making? Certainly in relation to Achilles tendon and ACL injury predisposition, there will be considerable challenges in interpreting the data and applying them wisely. As September et al. remark:

> The test results need to be interpreted in relation to the phenotype being a complex multifactorial clinical condition. It is therefore imperative that genetic testing not be offered directly to the public [DTC] but rather be used as a clinical tool requested by a referring health care professional.
>
> *(September et al. 2012)*

We have noted above how problematic the use of DTC genetic tests is in relation to concussions and trauma-related brain injury (Section 2.3). We shall explore this and further problems of DTC testing and predictability in the following chapter.

2.6 Genetic testing for developing tailored training programmes

Claude Bouchard's pioneering genetic experiments in the early 1980s (already mentioned in Chapter 1 in relation to the HERITAGE studies) have been essential to our understanding of human variability in response to exercise training. For more than 30 years his laboratory has studied inter-individual differences in response to training, or trainability. Common indicators of trainability are maximal oxygen uptake (V02 max), submaximal exercise capacity and adipose tissue mobilisation. The HERITAGE Family Study mentioned in Chapter 1 is probably the most comprehensive study offering information on trainability. Conducted from 1992 to 2004, the study featured 742 healthy but sedentary subjects following a highly standardised, well-controlled, laboratory-based endurance training programme for 20 weeks (Bouchard 2012). This programme induced significant changes in V02, for example, in responsiveness of V02 max to exercise training, changes that were characterised by a strong familial aggregation, i.e. prevalence in family members. This heterogeneity has since been replicated and thus confirmed in other populations, acquiring hence robustness and confirming that there is a substantial genetic component in trainability.

Over the past 30 years genetic scientists have not made much progress concerning precisely what genes are involved in response to training. This should not be surprising as trainability is a complex trait. What we know thanks to genome-wide linkage studies (GWLS) is that there are two loci, respectively one on chromosome 10p11 and one on chromosome 2q33.3-q34, that have been linked to training-induced changes in submaximal exercise. Some of the candidate genes belong to members of the kinesin family (which makes sense, as kinesins are motor protein involved in cellular transport, including the transport of chromosomes during mitosis and meiosis, neurotransmitters and other important 'molecular cargo': Argyropoulos et al. 2009). To conclude, we know that there is a genetic component to trainability but we do not know what genes are involved. Currently GWAS studies are under way (Ghosh et al. 2013). Other questions remain open, such as whether the response pattern in a given individual is specific to the given exercise mode and regimen, and whether the duration of the exercise intervention or training programme also makes a difference. It is plausible to speculate that there is a highly contextual response and that many genes are involved in trainability. For the moment it is impossible to predict from having certain allelic variations that somebody will a better response to an intervention.

2.7 Conclusions

There is a further set of concerns not raised here that we must record. One has to be very careful that when screening and testing is undertaken, associated ethical norms regarding commitment to confidentiality, privacy of information, duty of care to athlete patients and so on are observed. Counselling and education must accompany the data that these tests generate and it must be offered not only to athletes but to all athlete support personnel and coaches whose decisions shape the athletic well-being of those in their care (Juth and Munthe 2012).

As has often been said, neither screening nor testing on their own actually save lives, mitigate risk or enhance well-being. This is equally true of genetic testing. It is a tool, a means to an end, and it is only one tool. Other tools such as injury profiles, training regimes and educational programmes must have their place in informing policy and practice. Knowledge without wisdom can be a dangerous thing (Midgley 2002). As others have noted, the notion that SCT may bring about life-threatening incidents may be used to tailor specific training and performance profiles or it may be used to scare people away from exercising. Offering general advice is a dangerous game when one is unaware of the contexts in which the guidance will find its application. Likewise, understanding complex biomedical data is critical to appreciating risk. Neither are activities to be lightly undertaken. While coaches and athletic trainers are often quick to embrace performance-enhancing technologies, they are often slower off the mark to implement health protection measures. It is the job of sports scientists, policy developers, healthcare professionals and bioethicists to play their own role in these public debates. Nevertheless, while not embracing genetic reductionism, there will be policies, practices, rules and attitudes that can be shaped powerfully with greater genetic knowledge. Sorting out which and when is the key task if we are to ethically appraise their use wisely.

Notes

All websites accessed October 2017.

1 Part of the material contained in this chapter (Sections 2.2–2.5) was previously published in a different version in Camporesi, S., and M.J. McNamee. 2013. Is there a role for genetic testing in sports? In *Encyclopedia of Life Sciences*. Wiley Library Online, Chichester, UK: John Wiley & Sons, Ltd. We acknowledge Wiley for granting us permission to reprint.
2 One of us, Camporesi, had to undergo such screening when competing for her local track and field club in her hometown, Forlì, near Bologna, Italy, in the 1990s.
3 *Gillick v West Norfolk & Wisbech AHA & DHSS* [1983] 3 WLR (QBD)
4 www.publichealthdorset.org.uk/wp-content/uploads/2015/07/Fraser-Competencies-Guidance-and-Form-Smoking-Cessation.pdf. A similar court case was recently portrayed in Ian McEwan's novel *The Children Act* (2014), highlighting these tensions.
5 Thanks are expressed to Dr Matt Perry, Head of Medical Services of the English Premier League, for an insightful discussion of this issue, in relation to the duty of care of sports physicians.
6 At the proofreading stage of this volume we became aware that researchers at Boston University announced the development of a preliminary method of diagnosing CTE in living patients/athletes. This, if confirmed, could be a game-changer for the discussion on concussion-related traumatic brain injuries. See www.theringer.com/nfl/2017/9/27/16374868/boston-university-cte-research-breakthrough-player-fan-knowledge
7 The statement has since been taken off their website.
8 http://sports.espn.go.com/ncf/news/story?id=4293675
9 www.hematology.org/Advocacy/Statements/2650.aspx
10 www.hematology.org/Thehematologist/Features/1185.aspx

References

All websites accessed October 2017.

Abkowitz, J.L. 2013. Sickle cell trait and sports: is the NCAA a hematologist? *The Haemotologist*, 10(3). Available at: www.hematology.org/Thehematologist/President/1070.aspx

Anderson, L., D. Exeter and L. Bowyer. 2012. Sudden cardiac death: mandatory exclusion of athletes at risk is a step too far. *British Journal of Sports Medicine*, 46(5): 331–334.

Argyropoulos, G., A.M. Stütz, O. Ilnytska, T. Rice, M. Teran-Garcia, D.C. Rao ... and T. Rankinen. 2009. KIF5B gene sequence variation and response of cardiac stroke volume to regular exercise. *Physiological Genomics*, 36(2): 79–88.

Arneson, R.J. 1999. Human flourishing versus desire satisfaction. *Social Philosophy and Policy*, 16(1): 113–142.

Ashley-Koch, A., Q. Yang and R.S. Olney. 2000. Sickle hemoglobin (Hb S) allele and sickle cell disease: a HuGE review. *American Journal of Epidemiology*, 151(9): 839–845.

Bains, W. 2010. Genetic exceptionalism. *Nature Biotechnology*, 28(3): 212–213.

Berlin, I. (1969). *Four Essays on Liberty*. Oxford: Oxford University Press.

Bonham, V.L., G.J. Dover and L.C. Brody. 2010. Screening student athletes for sickle cell trait – a social and clinical experiment. *The New England Journal of Medicine*, 363(11): 997–999.

Bos, J.M., J.A. Towbin and M.J. Ackerman. 2009. Diagnostic, prognostic, and therapeutic implications of genetic testing for hypertrophic cardiomyopathy. *Journal of the American College of Cardiology*, 54(3): 201–211.

Bouchard, C. 2012. Genomic predictors of trainability. *Experimental Physiology*, 97(3): 347–352.

Collins, M. and M. Raleigh. 2009. Genetic risk factors for musculosketal soft tissue injuries. *Medicine Sport Science*, 54: 136–149.

Corlett, J.A. 2014. Should inter-collegiate football be eliminated? Assessing the arguments philosophically. *Sport, Ethics and Philosophy*, 8(2): 116–136.

Corrado, D., A. Pelliccia, H.H. Bjørnstad, L. Vanhees, A. Biffi, M. Borjesson and K.P. Mellwig. 2005. Cardiovascular pre-participation screening of young competitive athletes for prevention of sudden death: proposal for a common European protocol: consensus statement of the Study Group of Sport Cardiology of the Working Group of Cardiac Rehabilitation and Exercise Physiology and the Working Group of Myocardial and Pericardial Diseases of the European Society of Cardiology. *European Heart Journal*, 26(5): 516–524.

Culver, C.M. and B. Gert. 1982. *Philosophy in Medicine: Conceptual and Ethical Issues in Medicine and Psychiatry*. Oxford: Oxford University Press.

Dixon, N. 2001. Boxing, paternalism, and legal moralism. *Social Theory and Practice*, 27(2): 323–344.

Duncan, R.E., J. Savulescu, L. Gillam, R. Williamson and M.B. Delatycki. 2005. An international survey of predictive genetic testing in children for adult onset conditions. *Genetics in Medicine*, 7(6): 390–396.

Farioli, A., C.A. Christophi, C.C. Quarta and S.N. Kales. 2015. Incidence of sudden cardiac death in a young active population. *Journal of the American Heart Association*, 4(6): e001818.

Feinberg, J. 1986. *Harm to Self*. Oxford: Oxford University Press.

Gandy, S. and S.T. DeKosky. 2012. APOEε4 status and traumatic brain injury on the gridiron or the battlefield. *Science Translational Medicine*, 4(134): 134ed4.

Gavett, B.E., R.A. Stern and A.C. McKee. 2011. Chronic traumatic encephalopathy: a potential late effect of sport-related concussive and subconcussive head trauma. *Clinics in Sports Medicine*, 30(1): 179–188.

George, K.P., L.A. Wolfe and G.W. Burggraf. 1991. The 'athletic heart syndrome'. *Sports Medicine*, 11(5): 300–331.

Ghosh, S., J.C. Vivar, M.A. Sarzynski, Y. Sung, J.A. Timmons, C. Bouchard and T. Rankinen. 2013. Integrative pathway analysis of a genome-wide association study of VO2 max response to exercise training. *Journal of Applied Physiology*, 115(9): 1343–1359.

Goldberg, D.S. 2009. Concussions, professional sports, and conflicts of interest: why the National Football League's current policies are bad for its (players') health. *HEC Forum*, 20(4): 337–355. doi:10.1007/s10730–10008–9079–0

Goodlin, G.T., A.K. Roos, T.R. Roos, C. Hawkins, S. Beache, S. Baur and S.K. Kim. 2015. Applying personal genetic data to injury risk assessment in athletes. *PloS One*, 10(4): e0122676.

Halkin. A., A. Steinvil, R. Rosso et al. 2012. Preventing sudden death of athletes with electrocardiographic screening: what is the absolute benefit and how much will it cost? *Journal of the American College of Cardiology*, 60(22): 2271–2276. doi:10.1016/j.jacc.2012.09.003

Harmon, K.G., I.M. Asif, D. Klossner and J.A. Drezner. 2011. Incidence of sudden cardiac death in National Collegiate Athletic Association athletes. *Circulation*, 123(15): 1594–1600.

Hecht, A. 2002. Legal and ethical aspects of sports-related concussions: the Merril Hoge story. *Seton Hall Journal of Sport Law*, 12: 17–64.

Heggie, V. 2011. *A History of British Sports Medicine*. Manchester: Manchester University Press.

Holst, A.G., B.G. Winkel, J. Theilade, I.B. Kristensen, J.L. Thomsen, G.L. Ottesen and J. Tfelt-Hansen. 2010. Incidence and etiology of sports-related sudden cardiac death in Denmark – implications for preparticipation screening. *Heart Rhythm*, 7(10): 1365–1371.

Juth, N. and C. Munthe. 2012. Screening – how? In *The Ethics of Screening in Health Care and Medicine*. Netherlands: Springer.

Koo, S.H., C.S. Ku, P. Chui and E.J.D. Lee. 2011. Unravelling the mystery of sudden cardiac death through genetic approaches. In *Encyclopedia of Life Sciences*. Wiley Library Online. Chichester, UK: John Wiley & Sons, Ltd.

Lopez Frias, J.F. and M.J. McNamee. 2017. Ethics, brain injuries, and sports: prohibition, reform, and prudence. *Sport, Ethics and Philosophy*, 11(3): 1–17.

McCrory, P., W.H. Meeuwisse, M. Aubry, B. Cantu, J. Dvorak, R.J. Echemendia … and M. Turner. 2013. Consensus statement on concussion in sport: The 4th International Conference on Concussion in Sport held in Zurich, November 2012. *British Journal of Sports Medicine*, 47(5): 250–258.

McIntosh, A.S. and P. McCrory. 2005. Preventing head and neck injury. *British Journal of Sports Medicine*, 39(6): 314–318.

MacIntyre, D.A. 2016. 11 rules that made the NFL safer. *Wall Street Journal*. Available at: http://247wallst.com/healthcare-business/2016/11/06/11-rules-that-made-the-nfl-safer/

McKee, A.C., R.C. Cantu, C.J. Nowinski, E.T. Hedley-Whyte, B.E. Gavett, A.E. Budson … and R.A. Stern. 2009. Chronic traumatic encephalopathy in athletes: progressive tauopathy after repetitive head injury. *Journal of Neuropathology & Experimental Neurology*, 68(7): 709–735.

McNamee, M.J., B. Partridge and L. Anderson. 2015. Concussion in sport: conceptual and ethical issues. *Kinesiology Review*, 4(2): 190–202.

Marian, A.J., A. Mares Jr, D.P. Kelly, Q.T. Yu, A.B. Abchee, R. Hill and R. Roberts. 1995. Sudden cardiac death in hypertrophic cardiomyopathy. *European Heart Journal*, 16(3): 368–376.

Maron, B.J. 2002. Hypertrophic cardiomyopathy: a systematic review. *Jama*, 287(10): 1308–1320.

Midgley, M. 2002. *Wisdom, Information and Wonder: What is Knowledge For?* London: Routledge.

Mill, J.S. 1989 [orig. pub. 1859]. *On Liberty, with The Subjection of Women and Chapters on Socialism*, ed. S. Collini. Cambridge: Cambridge University Press.

Millspaugh, J.A. 1937. Dementia pugilistica. *US Naval Med Bull*, 35(297): e303.

Morgan, W.J. 2017. The ethical morass of college sports. In *Reflections on Ethics and Responsibility*. Munich, Germany: Springer International Publishing, pp. 117–133.

Myerson, M., M. Sanchez-Ross and M.V. Sherrid. 2012. Preparticipation athletic screening for genetic heart disease. *Progress in Cardiovascular Diseases*, 54(6): 543–552.

O'Connor, A. 2012. Should young athletes be screened for heart risk? *New York Times*, 30 April. Available at: http://well.blogs.nytimes.com/2012/04/30/heart-risk-in-athletes-is-gaining-attention/

Park, M. 2010. College football player who committed suicide had brain injury. *CNN News*. Available at: www.cnn.com/2010/HEALTH/09/14/thomas.football.brain/index.html

Partridge, B. 2014. Dazed and confused: sports medicine, conflicts of interest, and concussion management. *Journal of Bioethical Inquiry*, 11(1): 65–74.

Partridge, B. and W. Hall. 2014. Conflicts of interest in recommendations to use computerized neuropsychological tests to manage concussion in professional football codes. *Neuroethics*, 7(1): 63–74.

Pauling, L., H.A. Itano, S.J. Singer and I.C. Wells. 1949. Sickle cell anemia, a molecular disease. *American Association for the Advancement of Science*.

Pielke, R. 2016. *The Edge: The War against Cheating and Corruption in the Cutthroat World of Elite Sports*. Berkeley, CA: Roaring Forties Press.

Posthumus, M., M. Collins, J. Cook et al. 2010. Components of the transforming growth factor-β family and the pathogenesis of human Achilles tendon pathology – a genetic association study. *Rheumatology*, 49: 2090–2097.

Radford, C. 1988. Utilitarianism and the noble art. *Philosophy*, 63(243): 63–81.

Raikin, S.M., D.N. Garras and P.V. Krapchev. 2013. Achilles tendon injuries in a United States population. *Foot & Ankle International*, 34(4): 475–480.

Rees, D., T.N. Williams and M.T. Gladwin. 2010. Sickle-cell disease. *Lancet,* 376: 2018–2031.

Sailors, P.R. 2015. Personal foul: an evaluation of the moral status of football. *Journal of the Philosophy of Sport,* 42(2): 269–286.

Saulle, M. and B.D. Greenwald. 2012. Chronic traumatic encephalopathy: a review. *Rehabilitation Research and Practice,* 12: 1–9.

Savulescu, J. 2005. Compulsory genetic testing for APOE Epsilon 4 and boxing. In *Genetic Technology And Sport: Ethical Questions,* eds C.M. Tamburrini and T. Tännsjö. London: Routledge, pp. 136–146.

Scott, A., E. Huisman and K. Khan. 2011. Conservative treatment of chronic Achilles tendinopathy. *Canadian Medical Association Journal,* 183(10): 1159–1165.

September, A.V., M. Posthumus and M. Collins. 2012. Application of genomics in the prevention, treatment and management of Achilles tendinopathy and anterior cruciate ligament ruptures. *Recent Patents on DNA & Gene Sequences,* 6(3): 216–223.

Sovari, A.A., A.G. Kocheril and A.S. Baas. 2011. Sudden cardiac death. *Medscape Reference.* Available at: http://emedicine.medscape.com/article/151907-overview

Stein, R. 2010. Sickle cell testing of athletes stirs discrimination fears. *Washington Post.* Available at: www.washingtonpost.com/wp-dyn/content/article/2010/09/19/AR2010091904417.html

Tarini, B.A., M.A. Brooks and D.G. Bundy. 2012. A policy impact analysis of the mandatory NCAA sickle cell trait screening program. *Health Services Research,* 47(1pt2): 446–461.

Thomas, K. and B. Zarda. 2010. In N.C.A.A., question of bias over a test for a genetic trait. *The New York Times.* Available at: www.nytimes.com/2010/04/12/sports/12sickle.html

Thompson, P.D., R. Arena, D. Riebe and L.S. Pescatello. 2013. ACSM's new preparticipation health screening recommendations from ACSM's guidelines for exercise testing and prescription. *Current Sports Medicine Reports,* 12(4): 215–217.

Tsaras, G., A. Owusu-Ansah, F.O. Boateng and Y. Amoateng-Adjepong. 2009. Complications associated with sickle cell trait: a brief narrative review. *American Journal of Medicine,* 122(6): 507–512.

Verscaj, C., B. Abdolmohammadi, P. Kiernan, J. Chung, J. Crary, T. Stein … and J. Mez. 2017. APOE ε4 is a risk factor for chronic traumatic encephalopathy severity. *Neurology,* 88(16 Supplement): S9–1.

Vinocur, L. 2011. Sudden cardiac arrest kills too many young athletes. *Huffington Post.* Available at: www.huffingtonpost.com/leigh-vinocur-md/sudden-cardiac-death-_b_821483.html

Wheeler, R. 2006. Gillick or Fraser? A plea for consistency over competence in children. *British Medical Journal,* 332(7545): 807.

Williams, B. 1973. *Utilitarianism: For and Against,* with J.J.C. Smart. Cambridge: Cambridge University Press.

3

GENETIC TESTING FOR TALENT IDENTIFICATION AND DEVELOPMENT

3.1 Introduction: the future ain't what it used to be[1]

'The future ain't what it used to be' is a phrase widely attributed to the American baseball legend Yogi Berra, although it actually dates back to French poet and philosopher Paul Valéry, who wrote in 1937 that 'The future, like everything else, is no longer what it used to be' (Valéry 1937). Like all witticisms it contains a kernel of both humour and truthful insight. What was predicted as the future a few decades ago might be considered fanciful or timid according to the actual progress *inter alia* of science, technology and broader social trends. Moreover, aside from those who believe in fatalism, predestination or strict determinism, it is a matter of fact that our choices create new opportunities and close down others in *media res*; that is to say, in the thick of things. Life may be a noun, but living is a process, which unfolds before our eyes with more or less deference to what we would wish for. Randall (1939) writes that

> Our future is what we can *predict*; but what it *will be* in its actuality cannot be *foreseen* – at least by men. To say the future will be determinate now; though it will be what it will be, it *is* not *now* what it will be. This future that can be predicted from our present may be called the 'envisaged future'.

What these points amount to is at least this: guessing future acts, events and outcomes is a precarious affair. But predicting them is a far more hazardous affair perhaps best left to science-fiction writers. Some of the claims made by politicians, but often also by scientists and bioethicists, are unfortunately rather closer to science fiction than reality – such as claims that we would be able to defeat cancer by the early 2000s (US President Richard Nixon when he launched the 'War on Cancer' in 1971),[2] or the joint statement by former US President Bill Clinton with National

Institutes of Health Director Francis Collins and Celera Genomics CEO Craig Venter, at the 26 June 2000 announcement of the sequencing of the first draft of the human genome, that we would be able to benefit from the fruits of the Human Genome Project and unravel all the molecular basis of diseases in just a few years.[3]

As it should be evident from Chapter 1, we know very little about the genetic basis of sport performance. Studies ongoing since the late 1970s have identified only one allelic variant (the alfa-actinin 3 gene) which has been consistently and robustly associated with a specific performance phenotype: increased endurance. For all other alleles that have been identified as 'candidate genes', the study sample sizes have been too small; or other studies have failed to replicate the first findings; or we do not have animal studies to tell us the function of the protein in vivo.

3.2 What is 'talent' in sport?

Five factors play a major role in the development of athletic ability. These will be to a certain extent obvious to the reader, and are adopted and adapted from Yan et al. (2016):

a   *Deliberate practice*, operationally defined in the milestone study by Ericsson, Krampe and Tesch-Römer more than 25 years ago as 'engaging in activities created specifically to improve performance in a domain' (Ericsson et al. 1993).

b   *The role of the family in childhood*: parents/guardians obviously play a key role in the nurturing of any talent in children, not merely athletic talent. We unpack some of the ethical issues related to child-rearing and education below, and we outline how there is an inherent tension between the 'duties' of parents to help foster and development children's talents, and a possible breach of autonomy if parents end up fostering these talents in very aggressive ways.

c   *The role of coach and trainer*: in many ways the role of the coach/trainer is as pivotal as that of the family. Although similar, the two roles are not identical. For example, parents will have to have initiated their child to a particular sport before a coach can work on developing those skills or talents that the child may have. Often, the coach will 'take over' from the family in nurturing the child's talents. This will be in a best-case scenario, as there will also be those cases in which a child may be discouraged from pursuing a specific athletic career, for example because s/he has a slower development (see next point).

d   *Relative age effect*: it has been shown that individuals who are relatively older than their peers in a given cohort/year will perform better (Musch and Grondin 2001). These can lead to false positives (or, also, to false negatives for those children who develop relatively later) in talent identification and development programmes.

e   *Birthplace effect*: it goes without saying that it matters where we are born for the amount of opportunities that we may have (in sport, or any other context). The amount of opportunities available to children will vary tremendously depending on where they are born: without speaking about gross inequalities of access to training facilities and coaches between developing and developed countries, even in high-income countries there will be wide disparities between – say – the amount of training facilities available in the capital and in more provincial regions of the same country.

To offer an example of birthplace effect, let us take the case of a child growing up in a medium-size town of a high-income country (say, Italy) in the 1980s. The following were the sport activities available to the co-author as a girl: volleyball, soccer (football), basketball, tennis, swimming and athletics (track and field). If a child wanted to engage in, say, hockey or synchronised diving, the parents would have to drive the child at least one hour or two each day to the major city that would offer such facilities (Bologna, Milan or Rome), something not really feasible if both parents were working, even if they were committed to encouraging and nurturing their child's athletic abilities. Anecdotes aside, this example of a high-income country in the 1980s simply makes the point that it is not necessary to think about gross inequalities between countries to find examples of different degrees of opportunities for children related to the 'birthplace effect'. Yan et al. (2016) point to the absence of systematic data (qualitative and quantitative studies) linking the different factors that play a role in the development of athletic abilities, and point also at the lack of data exploring the contribution of each factor.

Talent identification is seen as an effective first step on the path to athletic success. On the basis of the results of these tests parents and coaches may identify, plan and invest in a child's future. However, the central concept of 'talent' is so complex that it is far from clearly mapped or universally agreed upon. In the literature on talent identification and development in sport the most widely cited text is Baker et al. (2013) who define talent as 'The quality (or qualities) identified at an earlier time that promotes (or predicts) exceptionality at a future time' (ibid., 3). Consistent with the above they refer to 'talent identification' as the 'Process of recognizing and selecting players, through a series of testing and subjective assessment procedures, who show potential to excel at a more advanced level of competition' (ibid., 5).

There are at least two conceptual problems with these definitions. The first is that their definition of talent does not track common linguistic usage. Thus, for example, the Oxford English Dictionary defines talent as a 'natural aptitude or skill', while Baker and co-authors define talent as a process. Second, Baker and co-authors link talent to future ability, as opposed to present ability. One could say that what they are referring to is potential talent, not talent per se.

In any case, Baker and co-authors rightly point out early in their work two problematic assumptions underpinning empirical research and applied practices in sport talent identification and development. The first of these assumptions is that talent is identifiable and quantifiable. The second is that adult performance can be predicted by earlier performance through specific 'markers' such as speed tests, power tests or genetic markers. This second assumption, translated to the field of genetic testing for talent identification, becomes that athletic excellence can be traced back to specific *genetic polymorphisms*.

Breitbach et al. (2014, 1493) identify a further problem when they note that the classification into 'talented', 'elite' or 'successful' athletes versus 'less-talented' or 'untalented', 'non-elite' or 'sub-elite' or 'unsuccessful' differs between different talent identification studies and depends most evidently on the availability of athlete groups for the studies – a point we have already noted in Chapter 1, where we also noted how classification depends also on the cultural and national context. They add that 'From a scientific perspective and for the purpose of TI, an appropriate definition of these performance classes remains necessary'. However, they also note how, that given the difficulties intrinsic in measuring something as complex as 'talent' in the first place, 'we seriously need to question whether any clear line can ever be drawn between talented, elite, successful and untalented, non-elite, unsuccessful athletes' (ibid., 1491). Hence this seems to be not only an empirical but also an epistemological problem. Importantly, they add: 'It seems like sports scientists are neither asking nor answering this question' (ibid.).

Because of all the aforementioned difficulties in defining talent, philosophical input is necessary when unpacking the scientific, epistemological and ethical issues inherent in talent identification in sport. There is an epistemological problem in the first place: talent is only something that can be identified with certainty in hindsight, while all the talent identification and development programmes are necessarily forward-looking. Profound as these epistemological challenges are, there are yet more – ethical – problems with these tests. A point that we make repeatedly in this volume is that ethical issues are often inextricably linked to epistemological issues in (genetic) science and technology. In the next section we discuss the former, before moving on to the latter.

3.3 DTC genetic testing for athletic talent: between science and hype

Direct-to-consumer (DTC) testing that provides analysis of genes in association with sports performance and sports talent is primarily based around the angiotensin I-converting enzyme (ACE) and the gene for α-actinin-3 (ACTN3). The ACE gene was the first to be widely recognised for its association with performance; in particular it was demonstrated to have an association with skeleto-muscle formation and function. In 2003 Yang and colleagues found that both male and female elite sprinters have a significantly higher frequency of the functional 477R genotype, where R stands in place of the amino acid arginine 'R' rather than a stop codon in the ACTN3 gene (Yang et al. 2003). Alfa-actinin belongs to a large family of actin-binding proteins, where actin is a fundamental component of the contractile unit of muscle fibres. Polymorphisms in ACTN3 are thought to contribute to the heritability of fibre-type distribution in muscle, where Type I muscle fibres are slow-twitch fibres that use aerobic metabolism and are used in endurance races, while Type II muscle fibres are fast-twitch fibres, which use anaerobic metabolism to create energy and are used in activities requiring short intense effort such as sprints or basketball, football and hockey (Berman and North 2010). Subsequent research has consistently supported the view that the genotypes of ACE and ACTN3 influence human performance in relation to sprint/power or endurance events. Although many genes and allelic variants have been tentatively associated with performance-related traits, these associations have not reached a conclusive level.

Webborn et al. (2015, 1488), surveying more than 40 DTC genetic testing companies noted that:

> Of the companies we identified, 54% of the companies offering DTC genetic tests related to exercise and sport do not publicly state which genetic variants they rely on. While commercial pressures undoubtedly exist, it is impossible for anyone – consumer, academic scholar or others – to scrutinise the service provided by the companies if the detail is not presented to the public.

In one of these companies, the test for 'ACTN3 Sports Gene' is sold as a genetic 'Power & Speed performance test'; the website of Atlas Sports Genetics at one point stated that its aim was to give 'parents and coaches early information on their child's genetic predisposition for success in team or individual speed/power or endurance sports'.[4] The same website also suggested that the results of the tests will be 'valuable in outlining training and conditioning programs necessary for athletic and sport development'. While the marketing strategies of DTC companies are not explicitly aimed at parents, the idea of exploring whether individuals are *inter alia* predisposed to athletic endeavours that variously require either endurance, speed or strength seems most effectively aimed towards children's unfolding capabilities.[5]

Aggressive marketing claims like those made by DTC companies often represent a clear overstatement of the predictive capabilities of genetic tests. There is also a general remark to be made about the wide discrepancy between the aim of research into genetics and sports, and the claims that these DTC companies typically make. On the one hand, the aim of research in genetics and sport is to identify the influence of genes within the performance environment, whether it is in determining risk of injuries or indicating predispositions to talent. On the other hand, we saw above an example of the far-fetched claims made by certain companies about the predictive power of their tests. This shift from experimental or therapeutic applications (i.e. the aim of research in genetics and sport) to enhancement intervention (i.e. the aim of the DTC genetic tests for athletic performance) must address substantial scientific problems, not least of all the extrapolation of data obtained under different experimental designs: to use the fact the results obtained on one pool of subjects (e.g. elite athletes in the case of ACTN3) are being applied to a completely different subset of individuals, i.e. children.

Caulfield (2011) argues that these tests are examples of the widespread phenomenon of the exploitation of science, or to use his neologism, 'scienceploitation', defined as the 'exploitation of legitimate fields of science and, too often, patients and the general public, for profit and personal gain' (ibid., 4). More recently, in 2017, Stephan Montgomery, a genetic scientist from Stanford, has launched a company which has quickly gone viral, called 'Except yes or no genomics'. This company mocks the claims of companies that work on a deterministic and reductionist understanding of biology and on the premise of genetic exceptionalism.[6] Let us consider whether the general public is being subjected to 'scienceploitation' in the case of the tests for ACTN3 variants. These tests claim to assess the predisposition to athletic ability and prowess, yet the ACTN3 gene accounts for only 2% of total variance in muscle performance (Eynon et al. 2011). Moreover, Lucia et al. (2007) report the single case study of a Spanish two-times Olympic world-class long-jumper whose achievements were especially significant because of the lack of ACTN3 gene expression in his sample. Thus it seems something of a leap to suggest that those who express the variant are better suited for sprints.

The bioethics and sports medicine community have taken a clear stance against irresponsible DTC marketing (McNamee et al. 2009; Camporesi 2013; Loland 2015; Camporesi and McNamee 2016). An Australian consensus statement on genetic testing in sport (Vlahovich et al. 2016, 4) states there is no scientific evidence for the predictive value of genetic profiling in sports performance, despite the correlation between some genes and elite athletic performance. In addition, a global group of experts has published a similar consensus statement clearly stating that there is no scientific basis for the use of genetic testing for talent identification and development in children (Webborn et al. 2015).

Notwithstanding the scientific consensus about the lack of evidence base for genetic testing for talent identification and development, the first study aiming at investigating the current use of, and attitudes towards, genetic testing in UK elite sport (Varley et al. 2018) found that although it is not commonplace, genetic testing does occur in UK elite sport, and that there is a widespread belief among support staff and elite athletes that genetics is an important factor in determining an athlete. Hence there is a willingness to engage in genetic testing to determine sport aptitude and injury susceptibility. The survey, which included multiple choice questions in addition to qualitative data in the form of additional comments, tested the attitudes and opinions of elite athletes and support staff at UK clubs for various sports and governing bodies in different contexts: current use, beliefs and potential utility of genetic testing in sport. The main findings of this first study were that the prevalence of the use of genetic testing within elite sport is low although not zero (14% of the elite athletes surveyed had previously engaged in genetic testing for sport performance, and 4% for injury susceptibility – with some discrepancy noted, as only respectively 2% and 5% of support staff reported such testing, potentially indicating that athletes do this on their own). The widespread belief, shared by scientific support staff and elite athletes, that genetics is important in determining athletic status, confirms the interest and curiosity of the British sport community in the potential use of genetic testing to determine aptitude towards certain types of sport, or response towards training, and to determine injury susceptibility.

Precisely how genetic testing should be used in the context of elite sport received mixed responses in the Varley et al. (2018) survey. There were issues of both specificity and sensitivity in the testing. Both scientific support staff and elite athletes mentioned more critically the possibility of missing unidentified or unidentifiable talent through genetic testing (false negatives) and also of producing false positive test results. They also raised the issue of possible genetic discrimination if athletes are selected out (not because they are false positive) on the basis of their genetic data. Views of support staff and athletes were mixed regarding this latter point, as while some noted that all athletes should be treated equally independently of the result of their genetic tests, others noted that professional athletes are routinely selected for employment according to different types of body measurement and performance capabilities, of which obviously genetic traits play a big part.

Hence, it seems that while extensive international discussions have taken place (Webborn et al. 2015; Vlahovich et al. 2016) regarding the use of genetic testing in children, these have not yet percolated into sport governing bodies and sport organisations regarding the wider potential for genetic testing: there is currently no guidance about how to ensure that genetic testing, when it occurs, is ethically justifiable and does not lead to discrimination or other unjust outcomes. As noted in the previous chapter, genetic testing used to screen for beta-thalassaemia could end up being discriminatory if African American athletes – who have a higher prevalence of the trait – end up being selected out – even if not formally somewhat informally – from participation in elite sport.

3.4 Regulating children's genetic testing: medical versus non-medical purposes?

Children, as legal minors, cannot lawfully give informed consent on procedures that *inter alia* require collection of their data (which includes tissue and other human samples). This is affirmed in law but also in a host of national and international treaties and policies. This general prohibition serves as the background for any discussion of genetic testing of children. Might there be exceptions to this position?

Specific to our present concerns it is noteworthy that the European Society of Human Genetics has recommended that testing in minors 'should be delayed until the person is old enough to make an informed choice' (Borry et al. 2009). Nevertheless, in a situation in which a minor is suspected to having a condition for which genetic testing may be clinically useful (for diagnostic or prognostic purposes), testing is generally understood to be a justifiable course of action, with parents acting as surrogate decision-makers for their child's informed consent. What, if any, latitude does this open up for our discussion of genetic testing for athletic talent in children?

Existing guidelines in Europe, such as the German Society of Human Genetics and the Danish Council for Ethics, have stressed that predictive and pre-symptomatic genetic testing during childhood or adolescence should only be performed for conditions for which preventive or therapeutic actions could and should be initiated (Borry et al. 2006). Their rationale, following the declaration of the World Medical Association, concerns the directness of benefits that research on and with children should bring to them as subjects of research. There has, however, been some loosening of this position by bodies such as the British Medical Association, and the Council for Organizations of Medical Sciences (CIOMS) (Edwards and McNamee 2005). In guidelines concerning research involving children,[7] CIOMS write:

> Before undertaking research involving children, the investigator must ensure that:
>
> - children will not be involved in research that might equally well be carried out with adults;
> - the purpose of the research is to obtain knowledge relevant to the health needs of children;
> - a parent or legal guardian of each child has given proxy consent;
> - the consent of each child has been obtained to the extent of the child's capabilities;
> - the child's refusal to participate in research must always be respected unless according to the research protocol the child would receive therapy for which there is no medically-acceptable alternative;
> - the risk presented by interventions not intended to benefit the individual child-subject is low and commensurate with the importance of the knowledge to be gained; and
> - interventions that are intended to provide therapeutic benefit are likely to be at least as advantageous to the individual child-subject as any available alternative.

With respect to testing, one must first settle the conceptual issue of whether indeed this is properly to be thought of as research. Insofar as it is, then the issue concerning the timing of the testing is apposite. There seems to be little point in testing for athletic potential during adulthood, given the trend for ever younger elite athlete status, and the need for early specialisation to become a successful athlete. However, as empirical studies have shown, the motivations that people have for ordering DTC genetic tests go well beyond clinical utility: what users 'get out of' DTC genetic testing has little, if anything, to do with clinical decision-making (Turrini 2015; Turrini and Prainsack 2016).

As a matter of fact, people order DTC genetic tests for a variety of motivations that mirror what they perceive as multiple 'utilities' of the tests based on their preferences and values. DTC genetic tests can also be 'identity-making': genomic information has been used to construct 'auto-biologies', narrative descriptions of a person's own identity based on biological data (Harris et al. 2014). As French sociologist Turrini puts it:

> This 'paradoxical' superimposition of clinical uselessness and satisfaction lies at the heart of consumer Personal Genomics and serves here as the starting point to reconsider the meaning of healthcare, medicine and body from the DTC GT users' perspective.
>
> (Turrini 2015, 58)

However, when performed on children, and if the testing is not directly connected to health needs, then DTC tests fail the second requirement outlined by CIOMS in their guidelines on research involving children. The assent of the child must be recognised as sufficient for the decision at hand, and respected where refusal is proffered. This is not merely a bioethical or biomedical guideline but is enshrined in the 1989 United Nations Convention on the Rights of the Child.[8] In particular Article 12 addressed the right of the child to be heard:

1. States Parties shall assure to the child who is capable of forming his or her own views the right to express those views freely in all matters affecting the child, the views of the child being given due weight in accordance with the age and maturity of the child.
2. For this purpose the child shall in particular be provided the opportunity to be heard in any judicial and administrative proceedings affecting the child, either directly, or through a representative or an appropriate body, in a manner consistent with the procedural rules of national law.

Now it is absolutely clear that the major point of taking such a test is to make a determination regarding the potential avenues that a child's life might or might not take. So, despite the lack of clarity of the designation 'research', the scope of this right goes to the heart of the decision-making consequences of the test. That does not settle the matter, however, since the last CIOMS guideline opens a further query relevant to our concerns, i.e. how one would, prior to the test, conceive of the benefits that it might confer. We shall return to this point in the conclusion of the chapter.

As with all international regulatory guidance, we find that it is more or less accepted in different states. For example, the German and Danish policies noted above retain their protective stands towards minors to a level beyond CIOMS guidance (Borry et al. 2006). Where there is not a strong diagnostic rationale for the testing (due to prevalence), it should be delayed until such time as the individuals to be tested have reached the age of majority or at least a level of competence.

The UK Human Genetics Commission and the Canadian College of Medical Genetics draw distinctions between 'medically significant genetic testing' (Canadian College)[9] and other tests that could have a 'significant or potentially detrimental impact on consumers' (UK Human Genetics Commission).[10] At first sight this does not look promising for genetically based talent testing. Moreover, genetic tests for predictive purposes such as talent identification for performance are potentially in breach of the Council of Europe Bioethics Convention article 12, as 'the idea of someone undergoing genetic testing in order to establish some kind of performance profile would itself go against the strict therapeutic or preventative rationale of the Council of Europe Convention' (McNamee et al. 2009, 341). The European Society of Human Genetics (ESHG) has also expressed concerns regarding the possibly inadequate consent process through which individuals are enrolled in research conducted by DTC companies with their samples or data. Perhaps against the tide of scholarly literature, the ESHG recommends that a separate consent procedure from the consent procedure for research should be implemented (ESHG 2010).

Caulfield et al. (2015) first considered the ethical issues raised by genetic testing for 'recreational purposes' or 'life-style oriented' genetic testing through the lens of children and adolescents. They have noted that the paucity of critical policy attention to these types of tests, in contrast to health-related tests, can be explained on the basis that these tests 'cannot do much harm' and thus are likely to fall within what might be considered permissive CIOMS guidelines. Is an assumption of non-harm warranted? We turn now to a consideration of some of these DTC tests.

Two sets of recommendations endorsed by the American College of Medical Genetics (ACMG) and the American Academy of Pediatrics were released in 2013 regarding genetic testing in children. In their joint statements both academies strongly discourage the use of DTC testing in children because of 'lack of oversight on test content, accuracy, and interpretation' (Ross et al. 2013). The recommendations address two distinct but potentially overlapping contexts (Clayton et al. 2014): (a) testing children for an adult-onset disease running in the family (i.e. families at risk) for which there is no cure; and (b) dealing with incidental findings discovered when performing exome or genome sequencing for a specific clinical indication in children. The former set of recommendations takes the position that such predictive testing should not be performed, with rare and carefully considered exceptions when diagnostic uncertainty poses a significant psycho-social burden to the family. Note these guidelines did not address the issue of looking for such variants when children are being tested to address another clinical issue. The second set of recommendations addresses the case of a child who undergoes testing for a specific clinical indication (i.e. to diagnose a disorder in the child) using exome or genome sequencing; the laboratory should also analyse and interpret the child's genomic data looking for known pathogenic mutations for which preventive measures or treatments are available. Moreover, the recommendations state that while patients/parents have a right to refuse genetic testing, if they do authorise it, they should not be given the choice of opting out of analysis of known further pathogenic mutations.

The ethical justification for genetic testing in children seems therefore to be shifting from the right to an open future (Feinberg 1980) to a 'life prospectus' argument (Ruddick 1988) where the interests of the children are inextricably linked to the interests of the parents, and of the family.

3.5 What it means to be a 'good parent': between nurturing talent, and enhancing autonomy

American philosopher of science and bioethicist James Tabery, in his original work about the struggle to overcome the nature/nurture debate (Tabery 2014), addresses the issue of how genetic technologies have, in the context of reproduction, changed the meaning of 'parenting' itself. Genetic knowledge enables us to intervene in a child's environment and this has impact on some of the interactional traits of children: only some of their 'susceptibilities' will be actualised, depending on the environment they find themselves in. But what does such genetic information amount to? Does this mean we have a duty to intervene? Ought we be considered blameworthy if we do not? And how does parenting change now that we know that certain decisions a parent took were triggered not by a particular philosophy of parenting, but rather by information they had about the consequences of their action on the actualisation of their children's susceptibilities? These questions are relevant for our discussion of genetic testing in sport, and as Tabery argues in the context of sex-selection, that 'what parents really want … is the freedom to have the sort of parenting experience they desire' (ibid., 3).

American legal scholar John Robertson played a key role in early ethico-legal debates on the apparent right of freedom of procreative choices. In 2003, Robertson discussed the case of parents using genetic tests and Prenatal Genetic Diagnosis (PGD) to select children with 'perfect pitch'. The gene for the perfect pitch runs in an autosomal dominant pattern, even though it has not been identified yet (Robertson 2003, 464–466). Robertson imagines a future in which the gene has been identified, and where parents who have a strong interest in the musical abilities of their children may be willing to undergo *in vitro* fertilisation and PGD 'to ensure this foundation for musical ability in their child' (ibid., 465). The case discussed by Robertson remains a thought experiment for now, but it is not so far-fetched to resemble a science-fiction scenario. The question is whether this request should be accepted or denied, approved of or frowned upon. Robertson argues that it should be accepted on the basis of the following argument: since parents 'clearly have a right to instill or develop their child's musical ability after birth' (ibid., 465), they might therefore 'plausibly argue that they should have that right before birth as well'. But is this really the case? To what extent do parents have a right to instill and develop their children's musical ability? Do they have a right to do so from the age of three, four or five years old? Is it a matter of fact that putting talented children in music or sports programmes at the earliest possible age is necessary to maximise the particular option to excel in music or competitive sport? But if that is the case, how many hours a day, or a week, do parents have a right to impose musical exercises on their children? Do parents have a right to do so at the expense of children being 'children'? To understand the implications of experiencing childhood means at least in part to understand that there are temporal goods intrinsic to that time of life (Slote 1986). The goal of creating successful musicians or talents of any kind does not justify any and all means.

At first sight, the use of genetic technologies after birth would seem to be less controversial than the use of germ-line genome editing. After all, how much can genetic technologies really shape an already existing person? Also, do we not already grant a great degree of leeway to parents in deciding how to rear and educate their children? Parents can impose their religion, hobbies, choice of school and friends on their children, and go to great lengths to 'nurture' their children's talents – from submitting them to heavy training schedules, to hiring private teachers or tutors, to sending them to intensive summer camps, and so forth. While these practices are occasionally subjected to criticism for their strictness, it is generally accepted that it is permissible for parents to steer children even aggressively in a particular direction. Not only that, but in Western society it seems that parents whose children exhibit precocious talents are bestowed with a duty to nurture that talent, and would not be considered to be 'good parents' if they failed to do so.

3.6 Between parental duties and child-centred decision-making: Feinberg vs Ruddick

The precise nature of duties and rights of parents and children has spawned a considerable literature that goes beyond our present concerns.[11] Our focus here is more limited, though the argument we want to challenge in this section is analogous to the argument used to justify the use of genetic technologies to scout out children's athletic talents, i.e. whether it is admirable or even permissible for parents to 'help' their children in these ways. It seems to us that this parental quality of nurturing children's talents is something that admits of degrees. Nurturing, though, has its own threshold beyond which features of domination intrude. Therefore, instead of condoning new practices of talent-scouting and talent-nurturing on the basis of established child-rearing practices, we should question the latter through the light shed by the former. It is well known that there is no shortage of excessively competitive parental attitudes aimed at nurturing and developing children's talents. There are extreme cases such as the death of an informal referee at the hands of a uncontrollably zealous parent at a North American ice hockey game in which the children of both fathers were playing (Butterfield 2002). Such horrors are of course tragic, but not especially enlightening from an ethical point of view, since in most sports parenting, even the worst sports parenting never reaches this far. Articulating a consistent ethical approach would be a worthwhile goal. We can only start such a development here in relation to genetic science and its application.

Caulfield et al. identify an autonomy-related issue in the use of genetic testing for athletic ability:

> To the extent that the information from these tests limits a child's or adolescent's ability to make decisions that are consistent with their goals, however, there may nevertheless be an autonomy concern. This concern may be more pronounced in some tests, such as many of the athletically focused tests, which actually look for specific variants of a particular gene and have the potential to limit a child's ability to explore different sports and activities.
>
> (Caulfield et al. 2015, 14)

How we analyse the child–parent relationship has implications for the ethical analysis of genetic testing for talent identification and development programmes. Avoiding a strictly analytical presentation of rights and duties, Ruddick (1988) argues that child–parent relations are based on a number of different perspectives regarding the role of the parent: (1) to care/attend to children's needs; (2) to care/attend to children's developments; (3) to care/attend to children's life prospects (or a combination of these three). These perspectives about the role of parents in child-rearing and education entail complex and contested accounts of important moral concepts, such as autonomy, best interests and rights. Disentangling these concepts is far from easy, and there can be no theory-neutral account, i.e. adopting (implicitly or explicitly) one perspective entails an ethical commitment. In this section we juxtapose two of these perspectives: Feinberg's right to an open future, and Ruddick's life prospectus principle, and see how they play out in the context of genetic testing for talent identification and development.

Both Feinberg's right to an open future and Ruddick's life prospectus principle find their roots in a debate on individual freedoms grounded largely in the context of educational opportunities. Similarly what prompted Feinberg's discussion, a classic in liberal educational, legal and political philosophy, was a US Supreme Court decision that permitted the Amish community to end their children's public schooling at grade 8 (aged 14 years) before the end of compulsory schooling at grade 10 (aged 16 years). The key issue was whether parents should rightfully have the discretionary authority to determine their children's religious and cultural upbringing, against a pervasive cultural background that was hostile to their way of life:

> The State is not concerned with the maintenance of an education system as an end in itself; it is rather attempting to nurture and develop the human potential of its children, whether Amish or non-Amish: to expand their knowledge, broaden their sensibilities, kindle their imagination, foster a spirit of free inquiry, and increase their human understanding and tolerance ... A State has a legitimate interest not only in seeking to prepare them for the life style that they may later choose, or at least to provide them with an option other than the life they have led in the past.[12]

While a meta-ethical discussion of the kinds of rights children may have and the authority of them over parental freedoms is beyond the scope of the present work, it is noteworthy that this line between 14 and 16 years is a relatively small one. There are mature 14-year-olds and immature 16-year-olds. It was a separate case in Kansas, *State vs Garber* (Davis 1997), where an Amish family sought to prevent their child going to a state-approved school, which made clearer the point of denial or restriction of opportunities:

> The case against the exemption for the Amish must rest entirely on the rights of Amish children, which the state as *parens patriae* is sworn to protect. An education that renders a child fit for only one way of life forecloses irrevocably his other options ... [C]ritical life-decisions will have been made irreversibly for a person well before he reaches the age of full discretion when he should be expected, in a free society, to make them himself.

(Feinberg 1980, 132)

Within a liberal society, the notion of negative freedom is highly cherished. We value freedom from many things including state domination but also the domination of others. This is necessary if our powers for autonomy are to be exercised meaningfully. Of course, with children these powers are more limited, a point remarked upon by most philosophers from antiquity until the twentieth century. Yet the idea of a right to an open future (ROF) is not without criticisms. Might parental child-rearing with a view to an open future, loosely aimed at some 'smorgasbord' of activities, not also be detrimental to the promise of a child's particular talents (Munthe 2005)? Does ROF count against all forms of early specialisation, which are necessarily exclusionary because of opportunity costs? The idea of a neutral, non-committal openness to the future also fails to capture the palpable fact that some options are not equally valuable nor necessarily combinable or realisable at the same life stage, but that they may still be rationally evaluated (Holm and McNamee 2011). We note in passing, and in fairness to Feinberg, that he was not entirely unaware of these problems and recognised that 'the Child's options in respect to life circumstances and character will be substantially narrowed well before he is an adult' (Feinberg 1980, 146). But concerns about genetically motivated interventions can apply well before the age of partly maturing dispositions.

For present concerns, we must establish the extent to which genetic testing for athletic potential falls more closely to the decisions in *Yoder* or *Garber* since there is a clear point that the kind of irreversibility to which Feinberg alerts us above is not the case with respect to the parents who seek genetics tests to identify their progeny's athletic potential. The question then becomes one of the timing of the intervention. Analogously, we might ask whether the children themselves might make that decision at age 14 or 16 and thus engage with the test on their own terms. This is not, however, what is considered when genetic tests are entertained to identify such potential since they are thought to be most effective when performed early on in children's lives.

The right to an open future is a useful heuristic in the consideration of these and related issues. But more must be done to think through the application of that right and what kinds of duties it creates for parents or guardians. For there is also a broader concern, that ROF fails to capture the widely held view that child-rearing practices cannot avoid significant recognition of parental values. Other, more child-centric, philosophers have pushed this dimension of the problem more attentively.

While Feinberg's thesis arises from the philosophy of law, William Ruddick's 'life prospectus principle' (1988)[13] emanates broadly speaking from within the philosophy of education. Ruddick considers the goals of parenting and child-rearing in the context of a family. When developing this principle, Ruddick came up with the analogy of 'gardener' and 'guardian' when thinking about parents and the way they have to fill in the interests of their child. These metaphors, and ones like them, were much the rage in the early phases of progressive philosophy of education. Ruddick offers a relational argument concerning parenting and child-rearing since, as he argues, the interests of the child are always intertwined with those of the parents. According to the life prospectus principle (LPP), parents are allowed 'to foster life-prospects that may eliminate a number of alternatives, as well as blocking life-prospects that on reflection they think could never lead to lives for their children that they, the parents, could accept' (Ruddick 1988).

Ruddick's account is to be seen as a competitor to Feinberg in the sense that whereas Feinberg's account is aimed at option maximisation, his own account is one of a life prospectus principle. While neither are extremes on this continuum, Ruddick's position is more of middle way between a domineering model of parenting with a non-committal openness. Note that both share the same opposition. Both are aimed at preventing what Ruddick calls 'parental self-perpetuation'. Ruddick argues that parents are required to provide life-prospects for their child(ren) that encompass a range of likely social circumstances that would sooner or later be acceptable to parent/child alike. He writes:

> The first condition requires parents to make informed predictions, for example, about social and economic circumstances that will define a child's occupational and other social possibilities and rewards many years hence. The second condition requires them to make similar long-range assessments of what they and their child will find an acceptable life for the child, then an adult.
>
> *(Ruddick 1988)*

One can see the attraction of this alternative to an excessively plastic account which Feinberg's ROF seems to assume. Yet the epistemic burden of reliably predicting the future seems excessive. Note also that genetic testing – far from foreclosing options – might if carefully handled assist in a flexible approach to decision-making by adding information to the subjective capacities of parents. This latter possibility would be conditional, however, upon the accuracy of such tests. And we have already questioned the efficacy of such above. Moreover, the tests ignore the complex interaction of genotype and phenotype (Tabery 2014; Loland 2015). Moreover, in so far as these were set aside there would still be the problem of access to valid interpretations of the tests themselves.

It would seem at first sight that the LPP could be used to justify exclusion of certain life prospects, but less so to justify actively pursuing some particular life prospects. One important point, raised by Ruddick and other child-centred theorists, is that parents not only raise children, but also create and sustain families with and for those children, a point worth considering when analysing benefits and opportunity costs of pursuing talent identification and development programmes. Feinberg's famous principle seems an unlikely support to genetic testing given that it seeks to prevent the narrowing of the life of the child. Ruddick's less familiar principle shares the feature of non-option narrowing, but despite its relational child-friendliness, it seems to place an epistemic burden that genetic tests, even if they were more predictively capable, could scarcely sustain.

A rights framework can help us think through some of the thorny issues. The 1989 UN Convention of the Rights of the Child has 41 articles. They vary in scope and function. We have noted above how Article 12 – the right to be heard – has application in our present discussion. But the kind of right that it is was not discussed. Many of the rights are protective of the welfare and interest of the child and are sometimes referred to as protective rights. Wall (2010) calls these top-down protection rights and bottom-up participation rights. Their sense is fairly obvious. Feinberg's thesis can be allocated the protective mode. In the case of zealous sports parenting, the use of genetic testing may be envisaged as occurring within a narrative of parental choice or even domination. Wall writes:

> Protection rights should identify those protected as … vulnerable. They should call for one another's responsiveness to difference. Not to be abused or exploited means not to be reduced to others' narratives and powers, not to be denied a particular social creativity of one's own.
>
> *(Wall 2010, 127)*

The latter point – non-subjection to the narratives of parents – seems to be the most apt description of the sports parents who live through the failures of their own sporting biography vicariously in the sought-for successes of their child's.

Ruddick is sensitive to the participation rights of children in so far as he acknowledges the relationality of child–parental decision-making and interests. But he fails to articulate a strong positive case. Wall goes further, after Eekelaar (1986), in articulating a kind of developmental provision right, embodying a position of children as neither passive nor autonomous. He rejects the dichotomy and attempts to articulate a dynamic interdependence between the parties. This looks like a solid model on which to build a developmentally respectful mode of relations between adults and children. What is less solid is the view that for the tests to be effective they must, most likely, be undertaken without the assent of the child whose voice and orientation are yet to be articulated.

3.7 Conclusions

We live in an era in which facts or evidence seem to be challenged by social-media-savvy sceptics. Why bother, then, that genetic tests devoid of scientific validity are being offered directly to the public so that parents, qua consumers, can make their own minds up in the race to shape their children's futures in a more or less consensual way? Caulfield and co-authors argue that:

> As many of the potential harms associated with these types of genetic tests pertain to a lack of accurate information and understanding about the validity and relevance of the genetic information provided, there may be a role for regulatory bodies responsible for enforcing truth in advertising standards.
>
> *(Caulfield et al. 2015, 17)*

A curb on these excesses is overdue, both in legal and professional terms. Genetic tests for talent identification purposes rest upon substantial assumptions about the envisaged future. This limitation is intrinsic to the prediction and not something that can be eradicated, since what one is predicting is, in part, the shape of a human life. What we do now affects the future for better or worse. And this is especially true of children and adolescents in the midst of their holistic development. Choices alter futures. None of this amounts to a conclusion that we should not use genetic tests, nor that we should. How we approach the initial question responsibly depends on our understanding of the terms of reference, the reliability and validity of the tests as they develop, and – crucially – a range of ethical considerations about choice, consent and responsibility for the future well-being of those whose life plans or prospectuses are neither fully formed nor informed.

In his complex work on personal identity and related philosophical concerns, Richard Wollheim opens by recalling an entry in Kierkegaard's *Journal* for the year 1843:

> It is perfectly true, as philosophers say, that life must be understood backwards. But they forget that other proposition, that it must be lived forwards. And if one thinks over that proposition it becomes more and more evident that life can never really be understood in time simply because at no particular moment can I find the necessary resting place from which to understand it–backwards.

> *(Wollheim 1984: 1)*

The extent to which genetic testing is used as a tool of enlightened choosing or systematic domination is rather like the Heideggerian point that technology is neither good nor bad in itself; it is a merely a tool for good and bad purposes. Knowing what we do about sports parenting, there may be good reasons for thinking not merely that it is more likely to be used as a domineering element of a controlling narrative, understood in a context of ever decreasing age in sporting specialisation and excellence. Latent prediction should not be wasted and so we must find out precisely and as early as possible what one is predisposed to in order effectively to fulfil potential. So goes the familiar story. There is a sense that this is precisely the kind of domination that Feinberg sought to protect against. Of course, the apparent paradox is that one cannot wait until the child has developed mature dispositions and can make informed choices regarding athletic careers if they are to excel. It will simply be too late. This of course does not mean parents must wait; indeed they cannot. Ruddick offers tangible advice and an appealing – though underworked – conceptual apparatus to justify this.

Genetic tests for athletic talent present scholars, scientists, policy-makers and practitioners (such as coaches) serious food for thought concerning the place of children in sports, but especially elite sports and talent development systems. A serious discussion needs to be opened on the meaning of sport and of physical activity in the child as compared to the meaning of sport in professional athletes. Sport in children should not (necessarily) be a 'goal-directed' activity aimed at victory or at pre-professionalising children, as elite sport is. The impact on the life of the children can be tremendous and cannot be justified in hindsight. This is at least part of Kierkegaard's point. When are we to fully appraise the value of our choices and those of our parents? Feinberg and others want to protect a space of opportunity; Eekelaar, Ruddick and Wall highlight the need for recognition of developing interdependence. While we wait for more insightful theory, perhaps it is best to warn against the zealous excesses of ill-founded biotechnological prediction.

At a non-genetic level, youth sports should not be framed exclusively as goal-directed activities (directed to victory). Sports at developmental levels must be understood differently from what it is for the professional athlete who is engaged in elite sport. The meaning of sport for the child must be pluriform: to stay healthy, to enjoy the company of friends, to enjoy the discovery of the possibilities of one's own body, to learn how to relate with a team, to learn the importance of rules and so on. It does not have to be, nor should it necessarily be, related to talent scouting and talent development.

Many philosophers of science and of ethics have railed against the elision of knowledge and wisdom. That we have the scientific knowledge and techniques or 'know-how' loosely to identify potential athletic talent does not lead to the conclusion that we ought to do so. Many phenotypic factors intervene between predisposition or potentiality and its actualisation. Not only are there costs to athletic success and failure, there are opportunity costs too – those paths to future selves and well-being that are occluded, closed down or simply not chosen.

Notes

All websites accessed October 2017.

1 The authors have been working on the topic for several years, and have published several articles (co-authored, or single-authored) on the topic. This chapter is substantially different from any of them, although naturally some of the ideas were developed for previous papers. The articles are: McNamee et al. (2009); Camporesi (2013); Webborn et al. (2015); Camporesi and McNamee (2016).
2 www.cancer.gov/about-nci/legislative/history/national-cancer-act-1971
3 www.genome.gov/10001356/june-2000-white-house-event/
4 www.atlasgene.com/
5 Although as an exception to the rule, the UK company DNAFit does not offer tests for under 18-year-olds.
6 www.frontlinegenomics.com/news/13369/scientists-fed-absurd-genetic-tests/#.WXR28 wb6Xyk.twitter
7 www.codex.vr.se/texts/international.html#children
8 www.ohchr.org/EN/ProfessionalInterest/Pages/CRC.aspx
9 https://ukgtn.nhs.uk/resources/library/article/human-genetics-commission-a-comm on-framework-of-principles-for-direct-to-consumer-genetic-testing-services-70/
10 www.ccmg-ccgm.org/documents/Policies_etc/Pos_Statements/PosStmt_EPP_DTC_ FINAL_20Jan2011.pdf
11 What we do not attempt, however, is a full-scale ethical analysis of the rights and duties of parents in relation to their children and their rights. Archard and Benatar (2010) lay out three variant positions from the parental package (parents get all rights but also all duties in toto); the no rights thesis (where they only have duties to children)

along with limited discretionary powers; and the priority thesis, (where rights are subordinate to duties).

12 *Wisconsin vs Yoder* et al., 406 US 205 (1972), 237–238.

13 An earlier form of Ruddick's position is laid out in his essay 'Parents and Life Prospects' (Ruddick 1979).

References

All websites accessed October 2017.

Archard, D. and D. Benatar. 2010. Introduction. In *Procreation and Parenthood*, eds D. Archard and D. Benatar. Oxford: Oxford University Press, pp. 1–29.

Ashley, E., N. Byrne, S. Camporesi, M. Collins and P. Dijkstra. 2015. Direct-to-consumer genetic testing for predicting sports performance and talent identification: consensus statement. *British Journal of Sports Medicine*, 49(23): 1486–1491.

Baker, J., S. Cobley and J. Schorer, eds. 2013. *Talent Identification and Development in Sport: International Perspectives*. London: Routledge.

Berman, Y. and K.N. North. 2010. A gene for speed: the emerging role of α-actinin-3 in muscle metabolism. *Physiology*, 25(4): 250–259.

Borry, P., L. Stultiëns, H. Nys, J.J. Cassiman and K. Dierickx. 2006. Presymptomatic and predictive genetic testing in minors: a systematic review of guidelines and position papers. *Clinical Genetics*, 70(5): 374–381.

Borry, P., G. Evers-Kiebooms, M.C. Cornel, A. Clarke and K. Dierickx. 2009. Genetic testing in asymptomatic minors: recommendations of the European Society of Human Genetics. *European Journal of Human Genetics*, 17(6): 720–721.

Breitbach, S., S. Tug and P. Simon. 2014. Conventional and genetic talent identification in sports: will recent developments trace talent? *Sports Medicine*, 44(11): 1489–1503.

Butterfield, F. 2002. Man convicted in fatal beating in dispute at son's hockey game. *The New York Times*. Available at: www.nytimes.com/2002/01/12/us/man-convicted-in-fatal-beating-in-dispute-at-son-s-hockey-game.html

Camporesi, S. 2013. Bend it like Beckham! The ethics of genetically testing children for athletic potential. *Sport, Ethics and Philosophy*, 7(2): 175–185.

Camporesi, S. and M.J. McNamee. 2016. Ethics, genetic testing, and athletic talent: children's best interests, and the right to an open (athletic) future. *Physiological Genomics*, 48(3): 191–195.

Caulfield, T. 2011. Predictive or preposterous? The marketing of DTC genetic testing. *Journal of Science Communication*, 10: 1–6.

Caulfield, T., P. Borry, M. Toews, B.S. Elger, H.T. Greely and A. McGuire. 2015. Marginally scientific? Genetic testing of children and adolescents for lifestyle and health promotion. *Journal of Law and the Biosciences*, 2(3): 627–644.

Clayton, E.W., L.B. McCullough, L.G. Biesecker, S. Joffe, L.F. Ross, S.M. Wolf, and For the Clinical Sequencing Exploratory Research (CSER) Consortium Pediatrics Working Group. 2014. Addressing the ethical challenges in genetic testing and sequencing of children. *The American Journal of Bioethics*, 14(3): 3–9.

Davis, D.S. 1997. The child's right to an open future: Yoder and beyond. *Cap. UL Rev.*, 26: 93–126.

Edwards, S.D. and M.J. McNamee. 2005. Ethical concerns regarding guidelines for the conduct of clinical research on children. *Journal of Medical Ethics*, 31(6): 351–354.

Eekelaar, J. 1986. The emergence of children's rights. *Oxford Journal of Legal Studies*, 6(2): 161–182.

Ericsson, K.A., R.T. Krampe and C. Tesch-Römer. 1993. The role of deliberate practice in the acquisition of expert performance. *Psychological Review*, 100(3): 363–406.

European Society of Human Genetics (ESHG). 2010. Statement of the ESHG on direct-to-consumer genetic testing for health-related purposes. *European Journal of Human Genetics*, 18(12): 1271.

Eynon, N., J.R. Ruiz, J. Oliveira, J.A. Duarte, R. Birk and A. Lucia. 2011. Genes and elite athletes: a roadmap for future research. *The Journal of Physiology*, 589(13): 3063–3070.

Feinberg, J. 1980. The child's right to an open future. In *Whose Child? Children's Rights, Parental Authority, and State Power*, eds W. Aiken and H. LaFollette. Totowa, NJ: Littlefield Adams Publisher.

Harris, A., S.E. Kelly and S. Wyatt. 2014. Autobiologies on YouTube: narratives of direct-to-consumer genetic testing. *New Genetics and Society*, 33(1): 60–78.

Holm, S. and M.J. McNamee. 2011. Physical enhancement: what baseline, whose judgment? In *Enhancing Human Capacities*, eds J. Savulescu, R. ter Meulen and G. Kahane. Oxford: John Wiley & Sons.

Loland, S. 2015. Against genetic tests for athletic talent: the primacy of the phenotype. *Sports Medicine*, 45(9): 1229–1233.

Lucia, A., J. Oliván, F. Gómez-Gallego, C. Santiago, M. Montil and C. Foster. 2007. Citius and longius (faster and longer) with no α-actinin-3 in skeletal muscles? *British Journal of Sports Medicine*, 41(9): 616–617.

McNamee, M.J., A. Müller, I. van Hilvoorde and S. Holm. 2009. Genetic testing and sports medicine ethics. *Sports Medicine*, 39(5): 339–344.

Munthe, C. 2005. Ethical aspects of controlling genetic doping. In *Genetic Technology and Sport*, eds T. Tännsjö and C. Tamburrini. Abingdon, UK: Routledge, pp. 107–125.

Musch, J. and S. Grondin. 2001. Unequal competition as an impediment to personal development: a review of the relative age effect in sport. *Developmental Review*, 21(2): 147–167.

Randall, J.H. Jnr. 1939. On understanding the history of philosophy. *Journal of Philosophy*, XXXVI (17 August): 460.

Robertson, J.A. 2003. Procreative liberty in the era of genomics. *Am. JL & Med.*, 29: 439–487.

Ross, L.F., H.M. Saal, R.R. Anderson and K.L. David. 2013. Ethical and policy issues in genetic testing and screening of children. *Pediatrics*, 131(3): 620–622.

Ruddick, W. 1979. Parents and life prospects. In *Having Children: Philosophical and Legal Reflections on Parenthood*, eds O. O'Neill and W. Ruddick. New York: Oxford University Press, pp. 123–137.

Ruddick, W. 1988. Parenthood: three concepts and a principle. In *Family Values: Issues in Ethics, Society and the Family*, ed. L.D. Houlgate. Belmont, CA: Wadsworth.

Slote, M. 1986. *Goods and Virtues*. Oxford: Clarendon Press.

Tabery, J. 2014. *Beyond Versus: The Struggle to Understand the Interaction of Nature and Nurture*. Cambridge, MA: MIT Press.

Turrini, M. 2015. Practicing the biomedicine to come: Direct-to-consumer genetic tests, healthism and beyond. *J. Med. Humanit. Soc. Stud. Sci. Technol*, 7(1–2).

Turrini, M. and B. Prainsack. 2016. Beyond clinical utility: the multiple values of DTC genetics. *Applied & Translational Genomics*, 8: 4–8.

Valéry, P. 1937. Our destiny and literature. In *Reflections on the World Today*, Pantheon Books, pp. 131–155.

Varley, I., S. Patel, A.G. Williams and P.J. Hennis. 2018, in press. The current use, and opinions of elite athletes and support staff in relation to genetic testing in elite sport within the UK. *Biology of Sport*.

Vlahovich, N., P.A. Fricker, M.A. Brown and D. Hughes. 2016. Ethics of genetic testing and research in sport: a position statement from the Australian Institute of Sport. *British Journal of Sports Medicine*, bjsports-2016.

Wall, J. 2010. *Ethics in Light of Childhood*. Washington, DC: Georgetown University Press.

Webborn, N., A. Williams, M. McNamee, C. Bouchard, Y. Pitsiladis, I. Ahmetov … and P. Dijkstra. 2015. Direct-to-consumer genetic testing for predicting sports performance and talent identification: Consensus statement. *British Journal of Sports Medicine*, 49(23): 1486–1491.

Wollheim, R. 1984. *The Thread of Life*. New Haven, CT: Yale University Press.

Yan, X., I. Papadimitriou, R. Lidor and N. Eynon. 2016. Nature versus nurture in determining athletic ability. *Medicine and Sport Science*, 61: 15–28.

Yang, N., D.G. MacArthur, J.P. Gulbin, A.G. Hahn, A.H. Beggs, S. Easteal and K. North. 2003. ACTN3 genotype is associated with human elite athletic performance. *The American Journal of Human Genetics*, 73(3): 627–631.

4

BIOBANKING IN SPORT: GOVERNANCE AND ETHICS

4.1 Introduction[1]

Biobanking sits at the intersection of many research disciplines and involves heterogeneous types of actors including legislators, policy-makers, research participants, researchers and funders. It raises issues of private and public interests, protection of individuals and the development of research that may have population-wide benefits. This complexity means that nuanced ethical and regulatory work is needed to provide quality governance and an ethically responsible environment for the conduct of sports genetic biobanking activities. In this chapter we first provide an overview of biobanking, commencing with an introduction to the nomenclature of the field. We then present some key epistemological issues and discuss the related ethical issues raised, i.e. privacy, security, ownership of data and informed consent. We use the Athlome Consortium[2] as the largest current example of collaborative sports genetic biobanking and discuss the tensions between individual rights and public benefits of genomic research as a critical ethical issue, particularly where benefits are less obvious, as in sports genomics.

4.2 Big data and biobanking: terminological clarifications

'Big data' is a phrase thrown around considerably in the media. But what does it actually mean? The first comprehensive and systematic meta-analysis of academic literature aimed at identifying the ethical issues of big data found that there is neither a commonly accepted definition of big data nor of biobanking shared across the literature, but that big data can refer both to the process and to the datasets themselves (Mittelstadt and Floridi 2016, 309). Biobanking by contrast has been with us for about 20 years. Biobanks are a generic name for a 'wide variety of methods and repositories for the collection of biological material' (Caulfield 2007, 211). The

World Medical Association defines biobanking rather blandly as a 'collection of biological material and associated data'.[3] Essentially they are storage resource sites comprising large-scale data (including tissue and other human samples) that can be combined for powerful statistical analyses on large-scale populations. The use of biobanks to store tissue or genetic material is not new *per se*, but the potentially global scale and combination of genotypic with phenotypic data is a recent development. It is this aspect that has generated new epistemological and normative challenges for researchers, clinicians and participants alike.

Although the purpose of 'research' is not included in the definition of biobanks, most of them are tied to specific research projects. Biobank research projects range from the disease-specific – for example, the Breast Cancer Campaign Tissue Bank – to population-scale – for example, UK Biobank – or to whole genome sequencing projects, such as the Harvard Personal Genome Project. Although they are often set up for prospective studies, they can also use existing sample collections, and are sometimes mixed (Henderson et al. 2013). There is a wide range of potential scientific and social benefits from such research, from how our genetic make-up interacts with environments, to drug targeting and sports performance. This heterogeneity raises many challenges for ethics and governance since a one-size-fits-all approach to biobanks may be insensitive to the specific needs of particular biobanks and their participants.

4.3 Epistemological issues in big data and biobanking research

The sheer complexity of the data (referring here both to the difficulty of analysing vast datasets and to the complex underlying algorithms) poses unique questions of comprehension not just for the general public but also for the experts. The epistemological issues of big data can be divided into two groups: issues related to a presumptive 'objectivity' of the data, and issues related to the context of the data. Referring to the former, data (like facts) are mistakenly said to 'speak for themselves'. Data are mistakenly treated as neutral and 'capable of explaining complex phenomena ... without need of further contextual knowledge, meaning, or interpretation' (Mittelstadt and Floridi 2016, 321). The idea of data-led 'objective' discoveries is problematic because it fails to recognise the role of the theoretical framework necessary to making sense of data that are in effect the outcome of complex processes and powerful assumptions. It is perhaps surprising that this very point was recognised 60 years ago in the philosophy of science, when the term 'theory ladenness of observation' (Hanson 1958) was coined. A part of the legacy of positivistic science, which assumed the categorical separation of fact and value in scientific operations, is still alive and kicking in much scientific research, as we also show in discussing the problems it brings in its wake in Chapter 10 in relation to the concept of race.

The reference to context relates to the second element of the complexity of big data. Too often the need to understand the context-driven meaning (or 'situatedness') of the data is dismissed by researchers when aggregating data for other uses.

Contextual features are typically stripped away and knowledge emerges from the data as a process of extrapolation irrespective of its (ir)relevance – as if the data had an existence somehow entirely separate from the context of their collection (Standish 2001). This is one of the flaws inherent in the process of aggregation of data, a process which often 'obscures the complex methodological decisions and ontological assumptions that ground the research that produced the data to be aggregated' (Mittelstadt and Floridi 2016, 321).

In 2016, the World Medical Association (WMA) published a three-page declaration intended to complement the Declaration of Helsinki (the cornerstone of clinical research ethics since 1964, now at its seventh revision (2013)), with 'additional principles for the ethical use of data in Health Database and human biological material in biobanks'. The declaration is addressed primarily to physicians and healthcare professionals and addresses mostly issues of informed consent, discussed in this chapter in Section 4.5. However, as some have noted (Aicardi et al. 2016; Lipworth et al. 2017), the scope of the declaration may be considered too narrow for the 'disruption' posed by digital data, which requires that knowledge and science as public goods are transparent, accessible and widely available. That is why some authors call for a more substantial revision of the rules and principles governing biomedical research, because of the unique epistemological challenges that reflect the need for a change in our ethical framework and language through which we express such ethical principles. We discuss one such substantial revision to the governance of biobanking in Section 4.8.

The blurring of traditional conceptual distinctions/dyads (health/non-health data; personal/non-personal data; individual/group-level privacy; primary/secondary uses of the data) in big data is important. As noted by Lipworth et al. (2017), these distinctions often form the basis of existing confidentiality/consent rules, which cease to be fit for purpose in the context of big data. The first important distinction that ceases to be valid in the context of big data and that is not addressed by the Declaration of Helsinki is the distinction between health and non-health data: Aicardi et al. (2016) note how many types of data can have some health connotation, even 'simple' web browsing data. Another definitional challenge is the distinction between personal and individual data, which is also not addressed by the declaration. Indeed, genetic information is 'personal' as it refers to the person, but is not exclusively to be thought of as 'individual', since genetic information reveals something about other persons involved (family, relatives). This has implications for the rights to privacy and self-determination that an individual may have over her own genetic information. Another epistemological/ethical issue identified by Lipworth et al. (2017) pertains to the return of data (result management/interpretation of results) and the responsibilities of researchers when encountering incidental findings. As noted by Woods, there is currently no international consensus on how findings should be managed, including incidental findings (Woods 2016). This is not an issue unique to biobanking research, but of course it is magnified exponentially by big data where the sheer volume of data increases the probability of incidental findings. The very meaning of 'incidental' in big data, one could say, is debatable.

What is incidental and what is not in research that does not have a clearly articulated theoretical question, but is 'data-driven'? Because of the absence of a clearly defined hypothesis, big data research operates in an environment which is much more likely to produce false positives, or spurious results, as identified by Ioannidis already in 2005.

Lipworth and co-authors also point out how some of the inherent technical and scientific concerns inherent in big data research, and the resulting epistemological misconceptions about the potential of big data, raise very concrete ethical questions, such as:

- possible harms to individuals, or groups of individuals, resulting from mis-predictions (from false positives);
- possible harms resulting from 'incidental findings' (for which some sort of protection should be in place);
- possible harms derived from obscuring the value-ladenness of data under the cloth of a presumptive objectivity of data-driven research;
- possible harms derived from over-hyping the benefits of this kind of research (to note, this is not by any means unique to big data, but is characteristic of genomics research, starting from the Human Genome Project), with, as a possible side effect, potentially stifling other kinds of research, and an under-mining of the trust of the public in science.

We agree with Lipworth et al. (2017) when they write: 'Because epistemology and ethics are so tightly linked in relation to big data, it is also the responsibility of scientists, research sponsors and peer reviewers to consider the complex epistemological issues raised by big data'. To note, the tight link between epistemology and ethics applies also to the context of research on race (see Chapter 10 in this volume).

4.4 Privacy, ownership and security of data

Privacy issues are frequently mentioned in conjunction with anonymisation and confidentiality, but they are distinct – even though of course there are overlaps. As pointed out by the Nuffield Council on Bioethics 2015 report on biological health data, the terms privacy and confidentiality are often used in conjunction or interchangeably, but should not be. In the definition they provide (Nuffield Council on Bioethics 2015, 50):

> Privacy concerns the interest people have in others' access to themselves, their homes and property, or to information about them. What counts as 'private' can change depending on social norms, the specific context, and the relationship between the person concerned and those who might enjoy access.

while:

> Confidentiality concerns the assurance that information provided by a person (or by another body) will not be further disclosed without their permission

(except in accordance with certain established laws, norms or expectations about when confidentiality obligations may be set aside).

The report adds that whereas privacy may be about access to several different things, confidentiality is exclusively about information. There is currently considerable confusion surrounding anonymisation of data. Elger and Caplan (2006, 662) cite 29 different descriptors for the degrees of anonymisation ranging from the identifiable to the unidentifiable. They include 'anonymised', 'completely anonymised', 'irretrievably unlinked to an identified person' and 'permanently de-linked'. It should be stressed how anonymisation of data in the big data era is extremely context- and time-dependent, i.e. what may be anonymous today may become re-identifiable tomorrow in light of technological advancement (Aicardi et al. 2016; Lipworth et al. 2017). As Aicardi et al. put it, 'Exemptions from research ethics requirements for supposedly anonymised data give the false and dangerous impression that anonymised data are inherently less prone to re-identification' (Aicardi et al. 2016, 210). A growing literature is building on the possibility of re-identification of anonymised data, and showing that while it may be possible to put in place some mechanisms to minimise this risk, this would inevitably entail the loss of valuable information in the process (valuable for research) (Sharon 2016; Lipworth et al. 2017). Not only that, but even if individual re-identification is protected through a sufficient aggregation of data, the potential for group discrimination (i.e. at the level of certain ethnic or minority groups) might still be possible. For present purposes, we simply observe the important terminological distinction between 'anonymous' referring to a status of data or material that was never identifiable to begin with, and anonymisation, which refers to the process through which something that was identifiable is made de-identifiable (Aicardi et al. 2016).

Another common triad often conflated in big data is that of *personal vs individual vs private data*, as already introduced in Section 4.3. Most if not all the data (understood as digital or analogic representation of biological samples) collected through biomedical research are personal data, as they pertain to the person. It should be noted, however, that not all personal data are individual (i.e. pertain only to the individual) and not all personal/individual data need to be thought of as private. Only a subset of personal data will be private data, i.e. data to which the individual does not wish others to have access (Nuffield Council on Bioethics 2015, 61). The distinction between personal and individual data in big data raises issues regarding rights to privacy and self-determination that an individual may have over her own genetic information, e.g. can there ever be a right to give broad consent when genetic information reveals information about others? Or can an individual have a right to communicate a result about her/his own genetic information to a relative when this result may have implications for the relative?

Broadly speaking, two types of measures exist to protect the interests of individuals against misuses of their data, the first one being types of operations that alter the data so that they can be de-identified (this pertains to the anonymisation of the data), and the second one that creates control on who has access to the data (this pertains to the ownership of the data) (Nuffield Council on Bioethics 2015). Data protection laws concern the processing of personal data, not privacy as such. In an effort to recognise all the nuances and contingency of the anonymisation process in big data, some scholars have developed contextual approaches to privacy, and argued that the expectations regarding privacy change depending on the context. For example, Nissenbaum (2011) has argued that depending on the nature of the context (medical, social or commercial) different norms regulate privacy. That makes intuitive sense, as information shared with one's doctor may not be the same as that shared with one's employer or work colleagues. However, the boundaries are not always that clear, and are increasingly being blurred, as it is the case for example for direct-to-consumer tests sold online. As pointed out by Prainsack (2017), all data can count as health data, and all data are potentially sensitive, depending on the context. A similar point regarding the context-sensitivity of what may be called personal data is made by McFee (2009) in the context of sports-related research, but the point is germane to all human data gathering.

4.5 Challenges to traditional consent models in biobanking

Biobanking research projects raise challenges to traditional forms of consent that have been widely accepted in medically related research for 50 years (Elger and Caplan, 2006). The consent process ordinarily takes place face to face and requires understanding of a specific protocol or study, in a specific time frame. Biobanking often fails, or does not attempt, to meet these standard requirements. Big data raise complications as individuals may be giving consent to the use of their data which is not only theirs, but also shared by family and relatives, including individuals not yet born, as DNA sequences may reveal probabilistic information about biological relatives, not only about the person from whom the sample was obtained. Hence new models of informed consent have been developed, which we discuss in detail below.

The first systematic attempt to standardise informed consent of an ethically justifiable kind in medical research arises from the Nuremberg Trial principles, and modified by the various Helsinki declarations of the World Medical Association, cited above. Two fundamental conceptual aspects of the traditional model of consent are voluntariness and informedness (Beauchamp 2011). Voluntariness refers to decisions made by potential participants free from coercion or undue influence, whereas informedness requires the decision-maker to have reasonably sufficient information in order to consent, or not. What does consent do? 'Consent sets aside norms and standards, such as the expectation of confidentiality, in specific ways for specific purposes. Consent does not abolish the underlying norm but modifies its application by creating a specific exception' (Nuffield Council on Bioethics 2015, 51).

The dominant norm for consent is written consent, where suitable surrogates are permissible for those without competence (Manson et al. 2007). First-person, written, informed consent has been seen as the 'gold standard' of clinical research. For research biobanks, however, which bring together existing data repositories, it is difficult or impossible to gain specific consent, as intended uses of the data were unknown at the time of joining. Not only might uses be unknown, but they may be in principle unknowable at any particular time in the ongoing research processes. A further problem arises in the contexts of retrospective or secondary-use consent. Many biobank collections contain samples taken with consent for a particular research use and stored accordingly following that use. There is no universal approach to consent for secondary uses, other than it should be broadly within original parameters and with research ethics committee oversight. The Public Population Project in Genomics and Society (P3G)[4] and Global Alliance for Genomics and Health (GA4GH) have developed guidance on assessing 'legacy collections' and consent which may assist Athlome in addressing the issue of re-use samples for international sharing.

Despite the widespread agreement about the general dimensions of consent (absence of coercion or undue influence; expected benefits, expected risks and safeguards; maintenance of privacy, anonymity and confidentiality; provision of verbal or written information regarding the project aims; right to withdraw without prejudice; and so on) it remains nevertheless a matter of interpretation to what constitutes a reasonable level of 'informedness', or when secondary or tertiary requests to participate are considered robust or coercive. For biobank ethics, informedness is a particular concern due to the highly complex nature of the research and the innovative methods involved. We have already discussed the unique epistemological challenges raised by biobanking in Section 4.3. There may be additional causes for concern if only a small number of people understand the systems and risks, and they are not the people explaining participation to donors. Fast moving, highly complex technology adds to the complexity of the ethical aspects of consent and governance more broadly. This can lead to reactive legislation, or defaulting to the most prescriptive applicable regulation where multiple jurisdictions apply (Laurie 2011). Under these conditions, a version of the precautionary principle may be applied that is disproportionate (O'Riordan and Cameron 1994) – i.e. more prohibitive than is strictly necessary for the purposes of protecting participants' interests.

Given that the first wave of bioethical research took the individual patient-clinician relationship as its paradigm, it is worth considering – in the light of biobank development – the extent to which this model is still fit for purpose. It is clear that there are some salient ethical differences between the traditional model of consent and the requirements of large-scale research processes that are more epidemiologically focused within a public health-oriented model (Dawson 2011; Holland 2007). Notwithstanding the norm for first-person written consent, in a primarily oral culture, or where there is no developed research governance, this may be problematic *inter alia* for reasons of trust. A global collaborative group such as Athlome, which conducts its research in a variety of institutions, will operate across a range of cultural norms. Therefore, it must include adaptive strategies for consent processes in order to reflect and respect differences plus adhere to agreed consortium-wide standards. Respect for international differences is especially important since there is a lack of population diversity in genetic biobank research (Haga 2009) and the facilitation of appropriate non-written consent processes may be one way to increase inclusivity.

Modern audio-video (AV) technology, being mobile and relatively cheap, has the potential to facilitate verbal consent in ways that do not undermine respect for persons within these cultures. Supporting information and updates can be sent to mobile technologies such as smartphones. Alternative means to facilitate verbal consent might be the use of voice over internet protocols and other audiovisual technologies. Guidance should be sought from the community, using local research ethics codes and procedures where they exist. This is particularly necessary with indigenous and other potentially vulnerable groups in the light of previous unethical conduct by researchers (Benatar and Brock 2011; Benatar and Singer 2010). It is paramount that local guidance ought always to be sought prior to beginning consent processes (Benatar and Brock 2011).

Even in the traditional model of consent, concerns remain as to whether participants are sufficiently informed and comprehend the known implications of engaging with research projects. For example, information may be given but not read, or read but not understood; care may or may not be taken with checking comprehension of what is being authorised. Manson et al. (2007) describe this as ritualisation of consent. If reduced to ritual, consent ceases to be meaningful and becomes merely a 'talisman' that serves principally to authorise research, absolving further duties or liability for researchers once it has been gained. Consent should instead be understood as a process rather than a single event (i.e. recording signature and date), a concept widely accepted in longitudinal research (Koenig 2014; Kaye et al. 2015). That consent should be understood as a process is a notion with serious implications for biobank research, given the promise of long-term storage and of potential new uses, questions and applications.

In addition to the challenges to informed consent we have noted, the populations from whom consent would be sought in the Athlome Consortium are not patients, who can be considered as highly motivated to participate in research, but healthy athletes. Those consenting to sequencing and/or secondary use of their previously collected samples may potentially uncover disease risk in themselves, or heritable traits that impact their families. This is not a risk that precludes non-clinical genomics, but requires pre-test counselling and considered reporting of results with further support where necessary. This burden on the participant without significant benefit to themselves or to their community may weaken the case for a move from informed to broad or other less stringent consent forms in the case of Athlome. These considerations lead us further to ask whether the traditional model of informed consent is even applicable to biobanks, a problem that has been widely discussed in the literature. The possible alternative models of consent to biobank research are discussed in the next section.

4.6 Evolutions of consent models for biobanking research

a) Blanket consent

Blanket consent arises when consent is sought and given for all types of research, or data uses, and no further permissions are sought further down the line. It is in effect a *carte blanche*. There is no specificity regarding use and no direct control by the participant over what types of research are carried out, including secondary uses of data. Of the consent models presented, blanket consent is the weakest in terms of protection of individual interests. It may have the property of voluntariness, but not of informedness. A participant retains the right to withdraw, but this is only useful if people know what research is being carried out to withdraw from. Practically, withdrawal is limited in biobanking, as once data is anonymised and de-linked it is extremely difficult to withdraw. The removal of a person or persons' information may have also a negative impact on other samples, as the power of large biobanks is in linking datasets on a large scale.

As the name suggests, blanket consent is non-specific and does not allow for the expression of specific preference. Caulfield argues there is no ethical justification to move towards blanket consent: 'The ad hoc modification of standard consent principles in favour of a blanket consent model undertaken in the name of near-future scientific goals, no matter how worthwhile, seems a dangerous path' (Caulfield 2007, 225). This is also the opinion of the WMA, stated in their recent 2016 declaration.

b) Open consent

Open consent was developed as a new model for consent within the context of the Personal Genome Project, led by Harvard pioneer George Church (Lunshof et al. 2008; Ball et al. 2014). According to the definition put forward by those who have developed it, open consent means that:

> volunteers consent to unrestricted redisclosure of data originating from a confidential relationship, namely their health records, and to unrestricted disclosure of information that emerges from any future research on their genotype-phenotype data set, the information content of which cannot be predicted. No promises of anonymity, privacy or confidentiality are made.
>
> *(Lunshof et al. 2008, 408–409)*

This unrestricted disclosure/redisclosure on the part of the subjects is premised upon a promise of veracity and trust on part of the researchers. The WMA in its 2016 declaration has deemed both blanket and open consent to be unethical, while leaving open the possibility of some forms of broad consent.

As stated by Article 19 of the WMA Declaration:

> An independent ethics committee must approve the establishment of Health Databases and Biobanks used for research and other purposes. In addition the ethics committee must approve use of data and biological material and check whether the consent given at the time of collection is sufficient for the planned use or if other measures have to be taken to protect the donor.

c) Broad consent

Broad consent is the model currently in use in many biobanks (Allen and Foulkes 2011; Master et al. 2012). UKBiobank, which houses over 500,000 samples, operates with broad consent and is supported in legislative terms by the Human Tissue Act in the UK. Broad consent can be described as consent to governance, rather than directly to research (Dawson 2011; Sheehan 2011). This represents a shift away from consent as the individual exercising control, or 'agent sovereignty' dependent on the specific project (Arneson 1999), to placing one's trust in a governing group and therefore giving control over to that group. In order to qualify as any kind of consent, it is argued that broad consent requires deliberation rather than just information, and as such can still respect personal autonomy via the considered choice to enter a biobank scheme and be governed (Dawson 2011). In broad consent a person agrees to an outline of research aims, with governance of research activities and dissemination of information to the public overseen by an appropriate governance committee, which should include participant members.

It is important to note how broad consent is not an antonym of consent (Nuffield Council on Bioethics 2015, 74) as it can cover a wide range of activities for specified purposes. In general, however, broad consent operates at a higher level of abstraction in contrast to more narrow consents, and usually refers to one-time consent for future research, in which each research use of samples and data must receive approval from an IRB (Institutional Review Board) or ethics committee (in this it differs from blanket consent). Despite its popularity with researchers who can use it for economic, efficiency and scientific gains, the broad consent model is not uncontroversial, and a few countries still prohibit the use of broad consent such as Germany, Mexico and South Africa (Rothstein et al. 2016).

d) Meta/tiered consent

Ploug and Holm (2015) propose a consent model that covers research uses throughout the course of a life. They call this 'meta consent'. Others, such as O'Doherty et al. (2011), Bunnik et al. (2013) and Rothstein et al. (2016), have referred to it as 'tiered' consent. Under this model of meta/tiered consent, specific types of research are consented to and can be amended over the life course at the discretion of the participant, with the justification that 'people should be given the opportunity to make choices based on their preferences for how and when to provide consent' (Ploug and Holm 2015, 5). Such a view places the possibility for a processual understanding of consent, but does not force it on the individual participant. Meta consent may protect participant autonomy by enabling a choice over the possible uses of data, which may be more or less specific. During the consent process participants are offered different options of types of research they can consent to. Usually it works with exclusion clauses (Rothstein et al. 2016, 166). Thus, for example, a participant may say 'yes' to cancer research, but 'no' to diabetes research. Equally, she may authorise use concerning one particular project (e.g. the UK Biobank breast cancer campaign tissue bank) but not others. Participants may also be invited to elect for their data to have unspecified future use. In a tiered consent approach, for instance, participants could be offered a menu of options pertaining to future research uses, request to re-consent, interest in returning results, or data sharing options (O'Doherty et al. 2011).

When participants are selective about the uses, they should be contacted when new directions or applications for the data are intended. One model for this re-contacting process is 'dynamic consent'.

e) Dynamic consent

Dynamic consent involves going back to the participant every time new use of data is proposed (Kaye et al. 2015) This reflects the 'gold standard' of informed consent per research project. It is not, however, without problems. Concerns include 'consent fatigue' due to repeated re-contacting, as well as placing an undue burden on participants for little or no personal benefit, for example, biobank research potentially benefiting future generations, but unlikely to have a direct (therapeutic) impact on those participating. This may affect both the numbers of people who sign up initially, and lead to higher attrition over the life of the research biobank. If consent becomes routine, it loses the quality that gives it validity in the first place (Ploug and Holm 2015). Other questions include how distinct the new use has to be from the original use consented to in order to need re-consent, and who decides the boundaries for this (Master et al. 2012). Dynamic consent could be utilised to facilitate a meta consent or broad consent approach. The consent sought on re-contacting might be broad or specific, depending on the context.

f) Waived consent

The Council for International Organisations of Medical Sciences (CIOMS) guidelines allow for waiver of informed consent requirement where risk is minimal. There are parallels here with policies of deemed consent for organ donation such as implemented in Wales from 2015, and sometimes, improperly, referred to as presumed consent. Since consent is an active verb, participants must give their consent. Insofar as it presumed, it is no longer consent. A point of contrast, however, is that the specifiability of the benefit from biobank research exists as a future potential.

Waived consent is less problematic in genomic research than in other practices such as organ procurement. However, this may be harder to justify for sports genomics, particularly for studies that are investigating genetic elements of elite performance, where there is a potential commercial gain, rather than say rare disease research, which has public health benefits. It could be argued that due to the intricate links between clinical research and, for example, pharmaceutical companies, all research is open to potential commercial profit. It is reasonable to suggest that any ethical framework should in part reflect the current norms of the society in which it operates. This can be challenging enough in one country, but becomes considerably more complex in international governance.

The right of participants to volunteer yet also withdraw their participation in research has been considered fundamental to ethical research conduct since the Nuremburg Trials. A recent challenge to this is the idea of moral obligation to take part in research; the future benefits to society being so great that not only is participating a contribution to the public good, but that those eligible have a moral duty to do so (Harris 2005; Rennie 2011). As with the move away from traditional informed consent, this seems harder to justify for sports than for other types of medical research where a direct benefit to clinical populations, as well as society more generally, can be established. In addition to the perceived differences between sports and clinical research in terms of obvious benefit, the moral duty to take part does not account for future-oriented genomics, but is concerned with more general medical research. It seems difficult to justify a moral obligation to participate in such open-ended future uses of biobank research information. However, as outlined in Section 4.4, it is unclear whether one can waive consent in the case of genomics research since the data often pertains not just to that individual, but also to family and relatives.

The European Society of Human Genetics suggests diversified informed consent. Consent is required where data are 'identifiable' and not where fully anonymised. There are concerns as to how complete any anonymisation or protection can be with improved technologies and increasing linkage of datasets. The complexity of anonymisation and linking technologies also has implication for the practical application of the right to withdraw. UK Biobank sets out tiers of withdrawal starting from 'no future use' to 'retain data' and to 'remove and destroy all data with no further contact'.[5] UK Biobank and others make explicit the fact that it will not be possible to remove data from existing or previous studies due to the measures taken to ensure privacy. The right to withdraw is therefore curtailed by the limits of technology and the ways in which the data are captured and used. The governance of datasets is not unified or harmonised in relation to the technologies of consented data.

The largest currently existing survey on participants' attitudes towards consent in biobanking is the study authored by Sanderson and co-authors in the US (Sanderson et al. 2017). The survey had 13,000 respondents and found 'no evidence to support the hypothesis that asking potential biobank participants to provide broad consent or permit open data sharing would lead to less willingness to participate than asking them to provide tiered consent or permit controlled data sharing' (Sanderson et al. 2017, 420), with the most endorsed benefit of participation the feeling of helping future generations, and the most endorsed concern a worry about privacy. Apple has been developing new models of consent including e-consent, which involves a two-step process in which participants (the users of some Apple app) are shown different kinds of textual and visual information regarding the study followed by a test aimed at assessing the comprehension of the material (note, this is also the model followed by 23&me) (Bot et al. 2016). The study shows that models of consent had little impact on patients' willingness to participate or not in biobank research. One of the factors that impacted the participants' decisions to participate was socio-demographic characteristics, e.g. minority groups such as African Americans were more sceptical about participation, being mindful of past research exploitations. Individuals with a lower level of education were also less likely to participate.

Having discussed the ethical challenges to genomic research biobanks, we now turn specifically to issues arising in the construction of the Athlome Consortium that will need to be addressed before it achieves its stated goals to 'collectively study the genotype and phenotype data currently available on elite athletes, in adaptation to exercise training (in both human and animal models) and on exercise-related musculoskeletal injuries from individual studies and from consortia worldwide' (Pitsiladis et al. 2016).

4.7 The Athlome Consortium

The drive to internationalise genetic biobanking is critical to its future success. As with any area of life, however, where there is a surfeit of laws, norms, codes and other regulatory codes, the difficulty is in knowing which one's research group or consortium should be guided by. In their review of best practices in biobanking Vaught and Lockhart claim that:

> Best practices have been developed by a number of leading national and international organisations … However the adoption of such practices is rarely well-coordinated, which has resulted in confusion over which practices are preferable or appropriate for particular biobanks or biobanking networks.
>
> *(Vaught and Lockhart 2012, 1573)*

The Athlome Project Consortium is an international research consortium bringing together separate researchers' projects aimed at studying genotype and phenotype data on elite athletes to understand the genetic basis of sport performance, the adaptive responses to exercise training and the genetic predisposition to injury. The Athlome Consortium is comprised of pre-existing Athlome projects that each act as a bio-guardian to protect the interests of participants in their specific project. It includes collaborative projects with research partners from countries in all developed regions of the world. Operating across six regions (Africa, Europe, Middle East, North America, Asia and Australasia), it raises regulatory and consent issues due to its global nature and due to the combining of existing cohorts or 'legacy collections' of genetic data that may long predate the consortium's existence.

As with all research consortia, ethical responsibility is distributed across the group. Each contributing element designates a researcher/clinician who is understood as a 'bio-guardian' (Pitsiladis et al. 2016). Additionally, the dynamics involved in consent for research, particularly at professional/elite level in sports, may raise additional concerns. The individual projects within the Athlome Consortium are, therefore, subject to a range of state, national and regional legislation and regulatory frameworks. Such frameworks originate in different jurisdictions and therefore reflect different cultural norms. What has been required as minimum consent in one country may not be the same as another. Regions include the EU, US and the UK, which have overarching data sharing laws such as the Data Protection Act, the European Data Protection Directive (due to come into force in 2018) and US Common Rule, but often do not have specific biobanking laws, as outlined in the review carried out by Rothstein et al. (2016). No universal data sharing treaty currently exists, but national laws and international guidelines have their basis in the Universal Declaration of Human Rights (UN General Assembly 1948, 217 (iii) A). Some countries differentiate between international sharing of samples and data; for example, in Taiwan sample sharing is not allowed at all, but data may be. Others may not differentiate explicitly, but have limitations on sharing; for example, in Denmark sharing is allowed with participant consent and a Danish collaborator (Rothstein et al. 2016). From a legal perspective, Mittelstadt and Floridi (2016) note how current data protection legislation in the USA (where we are witnessing an erosion of data protection laws, for example the 2008 Genetic Information Non Discrimination Act: de Paor 2017; Wauters and Van Hoyweghen 2016) may not be sufficient to protect participants from discrimination. That is why it becomes particularly important that institutional and ethics review boards, or consortium/ company review boards, play a role in developing guidelines to protect subjects where legislation is lacking.

In the Athlome Consortium, projects work across the regions mentioned, but also in areas where ethical and regulatory frameworks are less developed. It is a huge challenge to respect cultural norms and avoid imposing one dominant region's framework on to all partners, while protecting the interests of both the individual participant and the common interests of the research groups. The latest Council of Europe Recommendation (CM/Rec (2016) 6) places emphasis on interoperability and international cooperation in biobank research and gives some guidance on governance, oversight and transborder flows; for example, leaving open the methods by which this is to be achieved.[6]

Although much research in biobanks is prospective, existing samples may be used for new research purposes and may require retrospective consent. In retrospective studies, there is a likelihood of samples having been consented to using differing standards, or potentially not consented at all. Some retrospective biobanks may rely on 'old consent' from many years previous (Benatar and Brock 2011), which may not reflect the current thinking of the individual donor, and is unlikely to have included the uses now being proposed. This poses the question of how to ensure quality of consent while not impeding research due to the time and cost of procedures. The consent models discussed above may offer some recourse to the problem, but do not solve it. Where secondary research aims are not consistent with those for which consent was originally given, consent for the new uses should be gained, with the exception of fully anonymised materials (with the clause, noted above, that this may not always be possible). The secondary use of existing materials is a key challenge for Athlome and other similar collaborative projects; not only because of new uses, but also because of the differing standards and types of consent given by each partner's participants in the first place.

Collaboration brings rewards in terms of increased dataset size, diversity and analytical power, plus reduction in costs and need for replication. Yet with those rewards come challenges for consent and governance. Biobanks are governed by the legislative jurisdiction in which they are physically located. They may also be governed by regional legislation and governance frameworks, for example, EU Law, CIOMS, Council of Europe recommendations. Within a specific country there may also be state and federal legislation regarding data sharing and biobank research, for example, in the US and Germany. In the UK the Data Protection Act 1998 covers the whole union, but human tissue legislation operates differently with regard to consent for research using human tissue samples between Scotland and the rest of the UK,[7] leading to inconsistency in the law applicable to biobank research within the UK.

In 2013 the European Research Infrastructure Consortium (ERIC) for biobanking was established. This group develops standards for biobanks, but does not make significant contributions to addressing the 'diverse regulatory framework for biobanking in the EU and the Member States' (Reichel et al. 2014). Nevertheless, by definition, ERIC is limited in scope to Europe. Coalitions such as GA4GH and P3G have also produced instruments such as the Framework for Responsible Sharing of Genomic and Health-Related Data with the aim of providing means to ethically share data in a manner practical for all concerned (Global Alliance for Genomics and Health 2014). These offer a practical starting point for Athlome to develop governance to be tailored to its specific range of needs. While the EU makes law, and member states draw on such laws for their legislature, it is the responsibility of each member state to implement that law. Member states retain sovereignty both in the application of laws and in how they (states) relate to each other (Reichel et al. 2014). Frameworks such as ERIC's are closely tied to EU law, but the national law of the country in which a biobank is located will be the first legal control. This regulatory heterogeneity creates uncertainty, and is a barrier to effective collaboration (Mallette et al. 2013).

The complexity of sharing data across multiple unrelated jurisdictions, such as in the Athlome Consortium, is considerable. There is, therefore, a need to develop supporting ethical principles alongside a governance framework that encompasses and respects the differing norms of the countries involved. It is not appropriate to simply impose an existing legislation or framework on to the rest. Mallette et al. (2013) suggest a model governance framework that addresses some of the problems raised above, as part of P3G. The setting out of ethical principles, as opposed to a top-down prescriptive approach, aims to support common regulation by providing a shared base from which to develop more sophisticated governance. Proactively working to create foundational principles that guide law and governance can provide greater clarity and reduce the amount of reactive legislation necessary to catch up to technology. Athlome might be guided by the work of P3G, GA4GH, the TRUST Project, for example, in developing a central ethical framework that allows for international data sharing and sets out protocols for secondary use of samples and data. In doing so we must be careful to take a developmental approach, allowing flexibility to react quickly as needed and not 'create problems' in an attempt to be proactive. Operating with local codes and 'soft law' rather than through universal legislature may be a way to facilitate such an approach (Rothstein et al. 2016).

4.8 Beyond consent: solidarity and the governance of biobanks

As noted above, big data present some unique challenges to the traditional concept of informed consent, which requires understanding – and consenting to – participation in a single study, well defined in time and place, while big data by its very nature is 'intended by design to reveal unforeseen connections between data points' (Mittelstadt and Floridi 2016, 312), with the consequence that 'what the data reveals about the subject and its utility in future research present greater uncertainty than normal at the time of consent' (ibid.).

Prainsack and Buyx (2013; 2016) have developed a new approach to the governance of biobanks which goes beyond consent understood as individualistic authorisation. For them, biobank governance is really about the governance of risk and the governance through risk, and legal provisions in biobanking are aimed 'at minimizing risks such as access to identifiable information by unauthorized parties, discrimination or the accidental loss of data' (Prainsack and Buyx 2013, 73). Their innovative approach builds on their understanding of solidarity developed for a report commissioned by the Nuffield Council on Bioethics in 2011.[8] Prainsack and Buyx propose a shift from a dominant conception of individual autonomy towards a more social model, where harm mitigation strategies based on people's willingness to engage in activities that benefit others is the decisive aspect. They outline three tiers of solidarity: tier 1 works at the interpersonal level, where informal practices of solidarity emerge due a shared sense of similarity or shared causes. Tier 2 practices are also bottom-up but become formalised at the level of a community, while tier 3 practices are mandated/enforced by law or regulation. Their model is more sympathetic to biobanking governance where people engage in projects in which they are willing to donate time, bodily material, data (understood as the digital or analogue representation or biological matter) and information to contribute to research that can benefit others. This understanding is also based on increasing empirical evidence that shows that biobank participants are often willing to engage and let go of their privacy more than current autonomy-based governance allows (Aungst et al. 2017; Buyx et al. 2017). The relationship between participant and biobank is based on a relationship of trust that the biobank will hold up to its 'mission statement' or some other statement that provides insights into the 'value system of the biobank, which needs to be a mandatory part of any participatory agreement when the participants sign up to the biobank' (Prainsack and Buyx 2016, 81). (That is why a model of broad consent works well for a solidarity-based governance framework to biobanks.)

This approach is not without its critics. Woods (2016) has discussed some limitations of a solidarity approach to the governance of biobanks. He notes how a descriptive-only concept of solidarity, though it eschews the model of individual autonomy, inevitably includes other values (hence, it is not descriptive only). Thus when ethicists argue that solidarity should replace individual autonomy it is incumbent on them to articulate the moral load being taken on by that term. This presumption of group beneficence on the part of the researchers is context-dependent (Woods 2016). That means that, while it may be a valid assumption that people will freely and openly offer to donate samples in the context of the UK, where there is a national health system free at the point of delivery, it may not be a valid assumption for biobank research projects which operate within very different cultural contexts, for example in the US, or within private-led research projects, such as deCode Genetics (the Icelandic project aiming at sequencing the entirety of the Icelandic populations) or the *care.data* project, spearheaded by the UK government but privately led, to implement electronic health records access and sharing across the UK population.[9] The premise of the 'common good', and hence the willingness of participants to disclose or re-disclose their data, is highly context-dependent. Solidarity-based approaches work better when they are bottom-up, citizen-led, rather than top-down, government or privately led (Woods 2016).

4.9 Conclusion

While consent is only one of many ethical concerns around biobank research, it is undeniably a central one. We have here critically reviewed the main consent models either in use, or potentially appropriate for biobanking. For researchers, the more open the consent, the more potential research uses are available to be explored. Conversely, the more restricted the consent, the fewer possible uses without seeking further consent. With the exception of blanket and open consent forms, it seems clear that each of the consent types is viable on its own terms as part of an ethical model for biobank project development. The choice of consent model ought to some extent depend on, and reflect, the nature of the research being undertaken. Some flexibility seems unavoidable given that biobank development is in relative infancy compared with other forms of research programmes. It appears unjustifiable to prescribe too closely the forms of consent in such a rapidly developing and complex field.

Athlome and other collaborative sports genomics projects face challenges around collating data from previous projects. This should be done only where it is broadly consistent with the aims to which participants originally consented. Regulation is rendered extremely complex by the multiplicity of data sources, and it has been noted that a 'one size fits all' policy is a chimera in the case of international biobank or genomic research. While we have not discussed commercial uses of sports genomics data or the closure of biobanks, these are areas that merit further consideration, and should be part of any future framework. Fuller consideration of the other ethical concerns relating to biobank research should include reporting of results to participants (specifically incidental or secondary findings), deletion of data and the 'right to withdraw', and ownership of results and potential gains from results of research. Transparency and accountability as well as inclusive public engagement is vital from before the start of participant recruitment and continuing throughout the lifespan of a biobank or related research project.

These considerations should contribute to the nascent understanding of ethical and regulatory practices by considering how to meet the challenges of governance in the context of the Athlome Project and projects like it in the ethics of sports genomics, which is still in its infancy in comparison to medical or clinical ethics. For these reasons as well as those that apply to genomic research more generally, it is important that new biobank research groups such as Athlome embed robust ethical and regulatory practices in their structures from the outset. The careful consideration of underlying norms that inform how consent and other challenges for governance are conceptualised, and how data can be shared in a manner that is both ethical and supportive of the research, is key to developing and sustaining their success.

Notes

All websites accessed October 2017.

1 A version of Sections 4.5–4.7 of this chapter was previously published as 'Consent, ethics and genetic biobanks: the case of the Athlome project', *BMC Genomics* (2017, 18(Suppl 8):830 https://doi.org/10.1186/s12864-017-4189-1), co-authored by Rachel Thompson and Mike McNamee.
2 On a point of transparency, one author, McNamee, has assisted in varying degrees to the formation of the Athlome concept and project.
3 www.wma.net/policies-post/wma-declaration-of-taipei-on-ethical-considerations-regarding-health-databases-and-biobanks/
4 p3g.org
5 www.ukbiobank.ac.uk/
6 www.coe.int/en/web/freedom-expression/committee-of-ministers-adopted-texts/-/asset_publisher/aDXmrol0vvsU/content/recommendation-cm-rec-2016-1?_101_INSTANCE_aDXmrol0vvsU_viewMode=view/
7 On Scotland. See *Human Tissue Act (Scotland) 2006.* Elizabeth II. Edinburgh: Office of the Queen's Printer for Scotland; 2006.
8 http://nuffieldbioethics.org/project/solidarity
9 decode.com; care.data

References

All websites accessed October 2017.

Aicardi, C., L. Del Savio, E.S. Dove, F. Lucivero, N. Tempini and B. Prainsack. 2016. Emerging ethical issues regarding digital health data. On the World Medical Association Draft Declaration on Ethical Considerations Regarding Health Databases and Biobanks. *Croatian Medical Journal*, 57(2): 207–213.
Allen, C. and W.D. Foulkes. 2011. Qualitative thematic analysis of consent forms used in cancer genome sequencing. *BMC Medical Ethics*, 12(1): 14.

Arneson, R.J. 1999. Human flourishing versus desire satisfaction. *Social Philosophy and Policy*, 16(1): 113–142. Available from: doi:10.1017/S0265052500002272

Aungst, H., M.L. McGowan and J.R. Fishman. 2017. Participatory genomic research: ethical issues from the bottom up to the top down. *Annual Review of Genomics and Human Genetics*, 18: 357–367.

Ball, M.P., J.R. Bobe, M.F. Chou, T. Clegg, P.W. Estep, J.E. Lunshof ... and G.M. Church. 2014. Harvard Personal Genome Project: lessons from participatory public research. *Genome Medicine*, 6(2): 10.

Beauchamp, T.L. 2011. Informed consent: its history, meaning, and present challenges. *Cambridge Quarterly of Healthcare Ethics*, 20(4): 515–523.

Benatar, S. and G. Brock. 2011. *Global Health and Global Health Ethics*. Cambridge: Cambridge University Press.

Benatar, S. and P.A. Singer. 2010. Responsibilities in international research: a new look revisited. *Journal of Medical Ethics*, 36: 194–197.

Bot, B.M., C. Suver, E.C. Neto, M. Kellen, A. Klein, C. Bare ... and S.H. Friend. 2016. The mPower study, Parkinson disease mobile data collected using ResearchKit. *Scientific Data*, 3: 160011.

Bunnik, E.M., A.C.J. Janssens and M.H. Schermer. 2013. A tiered-layered-staged model for informed consent in personal genome testing. *European Journal of Human Genetics*, 21(6): 596–601.

Buyx, A., L. Del Savio, B. Prainsack and H. Völzke. 2017. Every participant is a PI. Citizen science and participatory governance in population studies. *International Journal of Epidemiology*, 46(2): 377–384.

Caulfield, T. 2007. Biobanks and blanket consent: the proper place of the public good and public perception rationales. *King's Law Journal*, 18(2): 209–226.

Dawson, A., ed. 2011. *Public Health Ethics: Key Concepts and Issues in Policy and Practice*. Cambridge: Cambridge University Press.

de Paor, A. 2017. Genetic discrimination: a case for a European legislative response? *European Journal of Health Law*, 24(2): 135–159.

Elger, B.S. and A.L. Caplan. 2006. Consent and anonymization in research involving biobanks. *EMBO Reports*, 7(7): 661–666.

Global Alliance for Genomics and Health. 2014. *Framework for Responsible Sharing of Genomic and Health-Related Data*. Available at: https://genomicsandhealth.org/about-the-global-alliance/key-documents/framework-responsible-sharing-genomic-and-health-related-data

Haga, S. 2009. Impact of limited population diversity of genome-wide association studies. *Genetics in Medicine*, 12(2): 81–84.

Hanson, N.R. 1958. *Patterns of Discovery*. Cambridge: Cambridge University Press.

Harris, J. 2005. Scientific research is a moral duty. *Journal of Medical Ethics*, 31(4): 242–248.

Henderson, G.E., R.J. Cadigan, T.P. Edwards, I. Conlon, A.G. Nelson, J.P. Evans ... and B.J. Weiner, 2013. Characterizing biobank organizations in the US: Results from a national survey. *Genome Medicine*, 5(1): 3.

Holland, S. 2007. *Public Health Ethics*. Cambridge: Polity.

Ioannidis, J.P. 2005. Why most published research findings are false. *PLoS Medicine*, 2(8): e124.

Kaye, J., E.A. Whitley, D. Lund, M. Morrison, H. Teare and K. Melham. 2015. Dynamic consent: a patient interface for twenty-first-century research networks. *European Journal of Human Genetics*, 23(2): 141–146.

Koenig, B. 2014. Have we asked too much of consent? *Hastings Center Report*, 44(4): 33–44.

Laurie, G. 2011. Reflexive governance in biobanking: On the value of policy led approaches and the need to recognise the limits of law. *Human Genetics*, 130(3): 347–356.

Lipworth, W., P.H. Mason, I. Kerridge and J.P. Ioannidis. 2017. Ethics and epistemology in big data research. *Journal of Bioethical Inquiry*: 1–12.

Lunshof, J.E., R. Chadwick, D.B. Vorhaus and G.M. Church. 2008. From genetic privacy to open consent. *Nature Reviews Genetics*, 9(5): 406–411.

McFee, G. 2009. *Ethics, Knowledge and Truth in Sports Research: An Epistemology of Sport*. London: Routledge.

Mallette, A., A.M. Tasse and B.M. Knoppers. 2013. *P3G Model Framework for Biobank Governance. Public Population Project in Genomics and Society (P3G)*. Available at: www. p3g.org/

Manson, N.C. and O. O'Neill. 2007. *Rethinking Informed Consent in Bioethics*. Cambridge: Cambridge University Press.

Master, Z., E. Nelson, B. Murdoch and T. Caulfield. 2012. Biobanks, consent and claims of consensus. *Nature Methods*, 9(9): 885–888.

Mittelstadt, B.D. and L. Floridi. 2016. The ethics of big data: current and foreseeable issues in biomedical contexts. In *The Ethics of Biomedical Big Data*, eds B.D. Mittelstadt and L. Floridi. Munich, Germany: Springer International Publishing, pp. 445–480.

Nissenbaum, H. 2011. A contextual approach to privacy online. *Daedalus*, 140(4): 32–48.

Nuffield Council on Bioethics. 2015. The collection, linking and use of data in biomedical research and health care: ethical issues. Available at: http://nuffieldbioethics.org/project/biological-health-data

O'Doherty, K.C., M.M. Burgess, K. Edwards, R.P. Gallagher, A.K. Hawkins, J. Kaye … and D.F. Winickoff. 2011. From consent to institutions: designing adaptive governance for genomic biobanks. *Social Science & Medicine*, 73(3): 367–374.

O'Riordan, T. and J. Cameron, eds. 1994. *Interpreting the Precautionary Principle*, vol. 2. Abingdon, Oxon: Earthscan.

Pitsiladis, Y.P., M. Tanaka, N. Eynon, C. Bouchard, K.N. North, A.G. Williams … and E. A. Ashley. 2016. Athlome Project Consortium: a concerted effort to discover genomic and other 'omic' markers of athletic performance. *Physiological Genomics*, 48(3): 183–190.

Ploug, T. and S. Holm. 2015. Meta consent: a flexible and autonomous way of obtaining informed consent for secondary research. *BMJ: British Medical Journal*, 350.

Prainsack, B. 2017. *Personalized Medicine: Empowered Patients in the 21st Century?* New York: NYU Press.

Prainsack, B. and A. Buyx. 2013. A solidarity-based approach to the governance of research biobanks. *Medical Law Review*, 21(1): 71–91.

Prainsack, B. and A. Buyx. 2016. *Solidarity in Biomedicine and Beyond*. Cambridge, UK: Cambridge University Press.

Reichel, J., A.S. Lind, M.G. Hansson and J.E. Litton. 2014. ERIC: a new governance tool for biobanking. *European Journal of Human Genetics*, 22: 1055–1057; doi:10.1038/ejhg.2014.6

Rennie, S. 2011. In whose interests? *Hastings Center Report*, 41(2): 40–47.

Rothstein, M.A., B.M. Knoppers and H.L. Harrell. 2016. Comparative approaches to biobanks and privacy. *The Journal of Law, Medicine & Ethics*, 44(1): 161–172.

Sanderson, S.C., K.B. Brothers, N.D. Mercaldo, E.W. Clayton, A.H.M. Antommaria, S.A. Aufox … and P. Conway. 2017. Public attitudes toward consent and data sharing in biobank research: a large multi-site experimental survey in the US. *The American Journal of Human Genetics*, 100(3): 414–427.

Sharon, T. 2016. The Googlization of health research: from disruptive innovation to disruptive ethics. *Personalized Medicine*, 13(6): 563–574.

Sheehan, M. 2011. Can broad consent be informed consent? *Public Health Ethics*, 4(3): 226–235.

Standish, P. 2001. Data return: the sense of the given in educational research. *Journal of Philosophy of Education*, 35(3): 497–518.

UN General Assembly. 1948. *Universal Declaration of Human Rights*. Paris: United Nations.

Vaught, J. and N.C. Lockhart. 2012. The evolution of biobanking best practices. *Clinica ChimicaAacta*, 413(19): 1569–1575.

Wauters, A. and I. Van Hoyweghen. 2016. Global trends on fears and concerns of genetic discrimination: a systematic literature review. *Journal of Human Genetics*, 61(4): 275–282.

Woods, S. 2016. Big data governance: solidarity and the patient voice. In *The Ethics of Biomedical Big Data*, eds B.D. Mittelstadt and L. Floridi. Munich, Germany: Springer International Publishing, pp. 221–238.

5

GENE TRANSFER, GENE ENHANCEMENT AND GENE DOPING: DISTINGUISHING SCIENCE FROM SCIENCE FICTION

5.1 Extending the tradition of medical self-experimentation: the case of BioViva[1]

Medical scientists have long used themselves as 'guinea pigs' for their own hypotheses. In the days before research governance existed in any robust sense we can see these pioneers, such as J.B.S. Haldane, as nobly wishing to avoid placing others under burdens that they wish to trial for safety. Take for example the case of Haldane. Here is how Harris (2009) reports it:

> Haldane wanted to build on work done by his father, John Scott Haldane, on the physiology of working Navy divers in the early 20th century. But whereas Haldane senior restricted himself to observation and measurement, his son took a more direct approach, repeatedly putting himself in a decompression chamber to investigate the physiological effects of various levels of gases. Haldane was motivated by concern for the welfare of sailors in disabled submarines, and his work led to a greatly improved understanding of nitrogen narcosis, as well as the safe use of various gases in breathing equipment. But he paid a high price, regularly experiencing seizures as a result of oxygen poisoning – one resulting in several crushed vertebrae.

In modern days, one suspects that the motives may be rather less laudable. One might even suspect researchers of deliberately trying to circumvent ethical and other norms and regulations designed to protect participants. An article in the *New Scientist* in 2016 reported that Elizabeth Parrish, CEO of the US-based anti-ageing biotechnology company BioViva, had become patient zero for two of the company's gene therapies (Le Page 2016). A further article provided additional details on the therapies: one is for follistatin, a myostatin inhibitor that is supposed to reverse muscle loss, while the other is for a gene therapy aimed at lengthening telomerases (Warmflash 2016). Telomerase are sequences of DNA at the end of chromosomes that get shorter every time a cell divides, and whose shortening is responsible for cellular ageing and senescence (Campisi and di Fagagna 2007; Shawi and Autexier 2008). A press-release from BioViva six months after the therapy supposedly showed Parrish's telomeres being 620 base pairs longer than in the previous measurement.[2]

In the US, the Food and Drug Administration (FDA) oversees the regulation of drugs through a highly regulated clinical trial system where drugs need to go through a three-step process before they are approved and enter the market. However, as we have argued elsewhere (Camporesi and McNamee 2014), sports are a highly specialised context where experimental participants (the athletes) have been shown to be willing to go to great lengths to try experimental unproven therapies on themselves, and where knowledge is not shared outside closed circles, e.g. teams, to maintain a competitive advantage. And then of course there are the East German athletes – properly thought of as 'subjects' – who were unwittingly subjected to a vast range of pioneering sports medicine techniques as part of the state-driven search for ideological supremacy via sporting success (Dimeo et al. 2011; Franke and Berendonk 1997; Hoberman 2001; Ungerleider 2001).

What BioViva's CEO Parrish is doing is in a sense circumventing traditional FDA regulations by trying drugs on herself as patient zero. Parrish explicitly said in an interview that she chose to bypass the FDA by trying the procedure overseas. The procedure took place in Colombia (Regalado 2015). Is Parrish to be praised as an heir to Haldane or indeed American surgeon William Stewart Halsted, who pioneered modern surgery by experimenting with anaesthetics on himself in the early twenty-first century? Or is she a reckless biotech CEO aiming to hit the media news with bogus therapies, or both? Parrish obviously sees herself as falling in the former category. In an interview challenging her on the ethical challenges of trying an experimental therapy on oneself without going through the FDA approval process, she responded: 'We as a company have our own ethics,' she says, referring to what she calls the need for inexpensive gene therapy treatments. 'I am certainly not going to ask someone's permission to potentially create new industries and cures' (Regalado 2015).

Parrish added: 'I am patient zero' and 'I have aging as a disease'.[3] There are many parallels between companies that aim to develop technologies to extend lifespan and to regenerate tissues, and possible applications in the context of sport. As a matter of fact, many of the gene therapy technologies that can be used to regenerate tissues after a stroke or infarction can also be used in the context of sport to enhance athletic potential. This dual use is a common phenomenon, not just in medicine but in many technological fields.

It comes as no surprise that Regalado (2015) reports 'BioViva is already getting calls from sportspeople desperate to try it themselves'. While there are yet to be confirmed cases of athletes using genetic technologies to enhance their bodies, athletes competing at the 2016 Rio Olympics were tested for 'gene doping' to increase EPO (erythropoietin) (Le Page 2016). The new test, developed by Australian molecular biologist Anna Baoutina, looked for added copies of the EPO gene, which stimulates the production of red blood cells (Baoutina et al. 2010). As is obvious, higher levels of red blood cells give endurance athletes an advantage in competition, assisting in speed endurance without actually adding to maximal levels of speed: it was thought to be the doping method of choice in the late 1990s and early 2000s in professional cycling. However, as some have noted, the test developed by Baoutina is only looking at one of the traditional targets of enhancement, i.e. increasing the number of red blood cells to improve oxygenation. There are many other targets of genetic technologies for which there is at present no clear test, while it may be plausible to think that detection tests could be developed to identify proteins like myostatin for which there are known mutations that increase muscle mass, or even proteins like vascular endothelial growth factor that increase oxygen carrying capacity, which is used in gene therapy after a stroke to improve muscle regeneration (Zentilin et al. 2010). Nevertheless, it would be much more difficult to develop tests aimed at assessing whether an athlete had had an 'infusion' of cells which have been engineered to increase an athlete's capacity for recovery, shortening the time needed to recuperate between training and thus allowing for greater intensity.

Before entering into the discussion of whether genetic technologies aimed at enhancing performance are to be considered as a form of innovation or a new form of doping, we analyse some feasible targets of the technology.

5.2 Targets of gene transfer to enhance athletic performance

Gene transfer aimed at enhancing athletic performance (gene enhancement, hereafter GE) employs the same techniques as those used in gene transfer for therapeutic purposes, which is referred to as gene therapy (GT) (Schneider and Friedmann 2006). Gene transfer is based on the delivery to a cell of a gene through a carrier. This can happen *ex vivo*, by withdrawing a human genetic sample, modifying it and re-implanting it into the patient, or more typically it is performed *in vivo* by direct delivery usually via a modified virus, but also a liposomic particle. The use of viruses as vectors to carry the genetically modified material has definite benefits, including the amount of material that can be conveyed and the duration of effects (Jager and Ehrhardt 2007). They are not without problems, though. Brzezianska et al. (2014) note irreversible side effects including unexpected virus recombinations, leading to the rapid transformation of normal cells and initiating tumours. We discuss these risks further in Section 5.3 in this chapter.

The aim of GT is to compensate for an absent or abnormally functioning gene. For sports enhancement, that would typically mean an intervention for the purpose of reinforcing muscular systems, increasing the number of red cells or increasing the threshold for pain in GE (a case discussed in detail in Chapter 7 in this volume). Gene transfer differs from other more traditional modes of doping insofar as, instead of administering the doping substance (e.g. erythropoietin, or EPO) to the athlete exogenously, a gene is administered to the body via a carrier, so that the body itself will produce EPO in higher quantities.

In line with one of the premises of this book, we are discussing only scientifically plausible scenarios, leaving aside bioethical discussions of science-fiction scenarios. The following are some of the most plausible targets for GE:

- Growth hormone (GH): has a multitude of effects on the body associated with growth, including a well-documented stimulatory effect on carbohydrate and fatty acid metabolism, and a possible anabolic effect on muscle proteins. Note that recombinant GH is already being used as a doping agent in sports (Baumann 2012).
- Insulin growth factor 1 (IGF-1): stimulates cellular proliferation, somatic growth and differentiation. In 1998, Dr Lee Sweeney (to note, now a member of WADA's Gene Doping Expert Group)[4] was the first to conduct *in vivo* gene transfer studies in mice using IGF-1 (Barton-Davis et al. 1998). The gene transfer successfully increased the strength of the mice, leading the press to dub them as 'Schwarzenegger mice' (Bartlett 2003). Macedo and co-authors created a mouse model of gene enhancement based on the AAV-mediated delivery of the IGF-1 cDNA to multiple muscles (Macedo et al. 2011). This treatment determined marked muscle hypertrophy, neovascularisation (growth of new blood vessels) and fast-to-slow fibre type transition, phenotypes similar to those experienced by athletes during endurance training. In functional terms, IGF-1-transferred mice showed impressive endurance gain, as determined by an exhaustive swimming test. The authors warned against the potential misuses of AAV-IGF1 as a doping agent as a 'realistic way to achieve a greater athletic performance' (ibid.).
- Myostatin: a protein that acts as a negative regulator of muscle mass. Mice in which the myostatin gene has been inactivated show marked muscle hypertrophy (Li et al. 2010) and a later report described similar muscle hypertrophy in a child carrying mutations in both copies of the myostatin gene (McFarlane et al. 2011). Therefore, the blockade of myostatin action has the potential to allow athletes to rapidly increase muscle mass.
- Erythropoietin (EPO): a glycoprotein produced by the kidney in response to a low oxygen concentration. EPO expression leads to an increase in red blood cell production and hence an increase in the blood's oxygen carrying capacity. EPO is one of the most widely used doping agents (Leuenberger et al. 2012).
- Vascular Endothelial Growth Factor (VEGF) and other angiogenic factors: their expression could improve microcirculation in muscle and hence increase oxygen and nutrient supply as well as removal of waste products (Wells 2008). There are already clinical trials under way or completed employing gene transfer techniques for angiogenesis purposes following an ischaemia (peripheral or of the heart). We discuss a case in point in Chapter 7 in this volume.
- Hypoxia-inducible factor 1 alpha (HIF-1-alpha): transcription factor activated under conditions of endurance exercise and muscle hypoxia, induces both the endogenous expression of EPO and VEGF. Consequently, increased expression

of HIF-1-alpha has the potential to substantially improve oxygen delivery to the skeletal and cardiac muscles (Borrione et al. 2008).

- Peroxisome-proliferator-activated receptor gamma (PPAR-gamma): the expression of the activated form of this protein in skeletal muscle increased the running endurance of transgenic mice to double that of wild-type littermates. Gene transfer of PPAR-gamma in athletes may improve endurance capacity by increasing the proportion of oxidative slow-twitch fibres (Østergård et al. 2005).

In attempting to ethically evaluate scientific and technological advances, it is important that scholars estimate responsibly what may be presently being attempted or what might be attempted in the near future. Long-term future gazing invites a form of speculation not always helpful to careful analysis and guidance. And this should be the stance of regulators who attempt to consider how to shape policy and practice responses to the threats and benefits such interventions may represent. We turn now to WADA's characterisation and regulatory framework for gene doping.

5.3 WADA's definition of gene doping and the precedents

As we will discuss in detail in the next chapter, contrary to what may be thought, the administration of substances with the aim to enhance athletic performance has not always been viewed with a negative connotation, but is instead a relatively recent development in the history of sport. WADA defines doping not as the ingestion of a performance-enhancing substance, but operationally as any form of anti-doping rule violation (WADA 2015). For our purposes, we focus on direct biological manipulation only. For a substance or method to be considered as doping and thus be included in the prohibited list, two of three criteria are currently necessary (i) [potential] performance enhancement; (ii) [potential] harm to health; and (iii) being contrary to the spirit of sport. How has WADA employed its methodology and criteria in relation to gene enhancement?

In 2001, shortly after the creation of WADA, the International Olympic Committee (IOC) convened the first working group on gene doping. The group's findings affirmed support for the medical application of gene therapy, but advised taking measures to keep genetic modification out of the realm of sports. Quoting from the official WADA publication, *Play True*:

> We endorse the development and application of gene therapy for the prevention and treatment of human disease. However, we are aware that there is the potential for abuse of gene therapy medicine and we shall begin to establish procedures and state-of-the-art testing methods for identifying athletes who might misuse such technology.

(Haisma and de Hon 2006)

In March 2002, the first workshop on gene doping was organised by WADA at the Banbury Center in New York.[5] Shortly thereafter, in 2004, WADA also created a Gene Doping Expert Group, with Theodore Friedmann as chair. Friedmann is the director of the Gene Therapy Lab at the University of California San Diego and a globally respected genetic scientist.

The IOC has inserted gene transfer technologies in its Prohibited List since 2003, under the umbrella heading of 'gene doping'. The most recent version of the Prohibited List (WADA 2017 version, page 5) as published by WADA contains the following proscription for Gene Doping:

> The following, with the potential to enhance sport performance, are prohibited:
>
> 1.   The transfer of polymers of nucleic acids or nucleic acid analogues;
> 2.   The use of normal or genetically modified cells. *(WADA 2017)*

This is a broad definition that aims at being inclusive of different types of genetically modified cells or nuclei acids (DNA/RNA). Gene doping is therefore defined by WADA to include the non-therapeutic use of genes, genetic elements or cells that have the potential to enhance athletic performance. It encompasses both gene and cellular therapy. WADA wants to make sure that all possibilities of gene or cellular transfer aimed at enhancing athletic performance are covered under the wide umbrella of 'gene doping'.

The first documented case of gene transfer aimed at enhancing athletic performance dates back to 2006 and took place in Germany. Thomas Springstein, track and field coach, was found guilty of trying to procure a gene transfer product called Repoxygen to administer to supposedly oblivious athletes. Repoxygen was a viral delivery vector carrying the human EPO gene under the control of a hypoxia response element, based on the principle of increasing the number of red cells in the athlete, and therefore of increasing their oxygen carrying capacity (Reynolds 2007; Fantz 2010). It was also an example of a direct bench-to-track-and-field transfer of technology, as Repoxygen was at that time being investigated in animal studies for a UK-based company called Oxford Biomedica. Therefore at that time there were no data at all on the effects and possible risks of the use of gene transfer for EPO in humans. As it will be evident now, even though gene doping had been included under the WADA Prohibited List in 2003, it is only since 2006 and the Repoxygen case in Germany that gene enhancement has become a documented reality to which regulators needed to respond.

Olivier Rabin, senior executive director at WADA, noted that the Repoxygen construct would have never allowed doping as there was an embedded turn-off promoter as soon as the animal was reaching a physiological level of haemoglobin concentration. He also noted that WADA investigated a few rumours in the past, all of which were related to the transfer of an extra copy of a gene (transgene) either related to EPO or to IGF-1 (Rabin, personal communication, July 2017).

5.4 Risks to health and challenges for detection

Gene enhancement techniques pose several risks to the health of the athlete that relate both to the kind of vector being employed (usually a modified virus), and to the encoded transgene (Harridge and Velloso 2008; Giacca and Zacchigna 2012; Brzezianska et al. 2014). As to the former, while gene transfer has proven relatively safe in clinical trials thus far (with some major exceptions, such as the death of 18-year-old clinical trial subject Jess Gelsinger due to immune-shock to the viral vector in 1998 (Lehrman 1999; Hollon 2000)), it is plausible to infer that gene enhancement, since it is not legally permissible, would be carried out in laboratories with less stringent regulations and greater health risks. Gene enhancement represents indeed an excellent example of technological determinism as discussed by Australian philosopher Nicholas Agar (Agar 2008). Agar refers to it as a 'catch-22': even if we deliberate that it is an ethically problematic technology, it is plausible to argue that 'somewhere else in the world', in some laboratories, techniques of gene transfer aimed at enhancing athletic performance in humans are being developed. However, we do not believe that this matter of fact should lead us to a 'catch-22'; quite on the contrary, it should encourage us to engage directly with the latest advancements in genetics and devise ethical ways to regulate them.

As to the latter risks (i.e. risks related to the encoded transgene), they are similar to those encountered in more traditional doping modes, but in addition both the level and the duration of protein expression are less amenable to control. For example, growth hormone and insulin-like growth factor 1 are both potent mitogen agents (i.e. stimulate cellular proliferation) and anti-apoptotic agents (i.e. inhibit physiological death mechanism). Both mechanisms, if de-regulated, can lead to an increased risk of oncogenesis (the development of tumour cells). Overexpression of EPO causes an increase in haematocrit, which in turn makes the blood more viscous and increases the load on the heart. Potential consequences include blockage of microcirculation, stroke and heart failure. In addition, the uncontrolled expression of the genes may in themselves be harmful. The production of viral vectors requires considerable purification and testing. Adenoviral vectors have been clearly associated with morbidity and in one case death after vascular administration in 1998, as mentioned above.

Gene transfer detection, though, poses unique challenges to detection. To start with, the protein produced through gene transfer will not be different in sequence or structure from the endogenously produced one. Anti-doping techniques aimed at identifying 'markers' of viral vectors have a low probability of success, as viral vectors may be measurable only shortly after administration, lowering therefore the probabilities of spotting them. In addition, detection would often require tissue sampling, as the administration of the vector would be performed directly into the muscular target tissue. Obviously, muscle biopsies are not an option for the athlete, therefore excluding this mode of detection (Baoutina et al. 2008). Alternative modes of detection called transcriptional profiling and aimed at detecting changes in protein levels compared to the physiologically measured basal level of the athlete would require simultaneous and repeated measuring of around 1,000 proteins (Rupert 2009; Reichel 2011).

As noted above, WADA runs a Gene and Cell Doping Expert Group chaired by Theodore Friedmann, which 'assists in establishing policies in the area of gene transfer in sport and in selecting research projects or programmes in genomics and proteomics'. WADA has actively been building a confident narrative around the possibility of detecting gene doping through 'sheer good-will' and generous funds.[6] Foreseeing a massive use of gene enhancement techniques in the London 2012 Olympics, WADA invested nearly $15 million to support research laboratories to develop methods for gene doping detection (*Business Standard* 2013). Among the funded laboratories was the Molecular Medicine-Gene Therapy laboratory at the International Genetic Centre for Genetic Engineering and Biotechnology, which received WADA funding to develop mouse models of genetic enhancement, such as the one mentioned above and developing mouse models of myostatin inhibited genes (Macedo et al. 2011), and subsequently to develop detection techniques.[7] In London, the King's College Drug Control Centre directed by David Cowan was appointed by WADA as the only UK laboratory responsible for gene doping detection and for 'championing Olympic integrity' at the 2012 London Olympics. King's College London later partnered up with a globally leading pharmaceutical company, GlaxoSmithKline, to enable its Drug Control Centre to operate a WADA-accredited satellite laboratory during the London 2012 Olympic and Paralympic Games.[8]

WADA former Director David Howman told the *Daily Telegraph* in 2010 that he was quite confident that gene enhancement strategies would be able to be detected.[9] In hindsight, his optimism seems over-confident. Indeed, any gene therapy product injected directly into the muscle will be very difficult to detect, as the expression of the gene product will be transient and detectable only through a muscle biopsy (rather than through a blood or urine test), which obviously is not a viable option for athletes given the potential for harm that the technique represents. As noted above, athlete biopsies are not permitted as means of detection (Fischetto and Bermon 2013; Aquino Neto et al. 2016). Moreover, gene editing techniques through the latest genome editing technology CRISPR may virtually be undetectable as they do not need any carrier, and allow targeted single-letter changes in genes which are indistinguishable from naturally occurring variations (Polcz and Lewis 2016). This all paints a somewhat less definitive picture of the possibilities for actual detection of genetic technologies used for enhancement.[10]

Neither the London 2012 nor the Rio 2016 Olympic Game witnessed the 'gene doping' scandals that had allegedly been presaged by the media or scholars beforehand (Miah 2004; Foddy and Savulescu 2007). There have been, though, speculations on Chinese swimmer Ye Shiwen, who won the 400 metres individual medley in London setting a new world record in 4 minutes 28 seconds, and swimming the last 100 metres faster than the male US swimmer Ryan Lochte in his individual gold-medal-winning time. This detail led to the public accusation by John Leonard, executive director of the World Swimming Coaches Association (USA office), that her victory was 'disturbing', and that she may have cheated. The British tabloid newspaper, the *Daily Mail*, pounced on the case and speculated about the possibility of genetic modification: 'The astonishing suggestion seems to be that London 2012 may be the first Olympics in which competitors are attempting to cheat by altering their genes to build muscle and sinew, and boost their blood's oxygen-carrying powers' (Naish 2012).

It is important to note that Shiwen later tested negative at the anti-doping control, and John Leonard had to deliver a public apology. The result of the anti-doping control did not quench completely, though, the speculations that China may have undertaken state-sponsored genetic modification experiments to breed athletes. The scenario, though science-fictional, is not too far from the documented reality of Chinese-based talent scout camps for very young children, where traditional modes of talent-scouting have been coupled with new genetic technologies to identify potential future Olympians.[11]

5.5 Gene transfer to enhance athletic performance: innovation or doping?

As we can read in the following statement published on WADA's official publication *Play True*, WADA considers gene transfer technologies aimed at enhancing athletic performance to be a form of doping:

> Gene doping represents a threat to the integrity of sport [c] and the health of athletes [b], and as the international organization responsible for promoting, coordinating and monitoring the global fight against doping in sport in all its forms, WADA is devoting significant resources and attention to ways that will enable the detection of gene doping.
>
> *(WADA 2008)*

Along similar lines, according to the Australian 2016 consensus statement,

> In the case of using gene therapy to treat serious conditions, the benefits of treatment often outweigh the risks. The use of genetic modification in the attempt to improve sporting performance, however, is unlikely to confer such a favourable benefit to risk ratio. It is unethical to attempt genetic modification on elite athletes with the aim of achieving performance gains.
>
> *(Vlahovich et al. 2016, 4)*

This view presupposes that attempting genetic modification is against the spirit of sport. However, this view is not universally shared by bioethicists and philosophers of sport.

The very act of labelling this type of genetic modification as 'doping' is a significant decision, clearly connoting an official negative attitude towards the practice. But ought gene transfer techniques be classified as doping? The play *Deny Deny* by Jonathan Maitland, shown at London's Park Theatre in 2016, depicts the story of a young athlete who, encouraged by her coach (interestingly, also a sports physician), decides to embark on a new experimental procedure in which cells of her body are collected, genetically engineered and administered back, with the explicit purpose of allowing her a faster recovery. The athlete asks: 'Is it legal?' The coach responds: 'Look into the Code and tell me if it is not.' The play does an excellent job at illustrating how the issue of gene doping is much more nuanced than how WADA paints it. Yet national and international policy frameworks are rarely inclined towards acknowledging complexity. Their first task is to deter what they determine deviant behaviour; their second is to educate; and their third will be to sanction non-compliant athletes (and now it seems, possibly states too).

Genetic engineering is an experimental new frontier of research, and according to the coach in *Deny Deny*, athletes experimenting on themselves should be considered pioneers (rather like Elizabeth Parrish's self-promoting narrative described at the beginning of this chapter) and praised, not blamed, for taking all the risks upon themselves in order to attain the desired rewards. Of course, such self-experimentations in the context of sport do not necessarily have as a primary motivation the advancement of knowledge in the medical field, and thus benefit to others. Athletes, and the entourages around them, do not want to lose the competitive advantage they hope to derive from these experimental therapies by sharing with fellow competitors the knowledge acquired experimenting on themselves (Camporesi 2017).

According to Andy Miah, author of the first full-length treatment of genetic modification in athletes, genetic enhancement and doping are 'quite different forms of performance enhancement that cannot be treated alike' (Miah 2004, 147). Miah views genetic enhancement as a form of innovation in sport, and he compares it to 'the development of fibreglass poles in pole vaulting, or Fosbury flop in high jump' (ibid., 160). In this sense Miah understands genetic enhancement as 'an innovation that enhances the capacity to express sports-related skills'. In his account, gene enhancement is not a permissive threat to the excellences inherent in sports, which is one of the arguments that have been put forward by philosophers to justify the continuing ban on doping (Devine 2010; Loland 2017; Murray 2009), but on the contrary genetic enhancement allows the pursuit of excellence in sport by allowing athletes to train longer and harder. This is also the view underlying *Deny Deny*, where the coach reassures the protagonist that she would not be cheating; simply the technology would provide her body with a way of recovering faster, and training for longer hours. It is only in this way that technology would provide the athlete with an advantage in competition.

Other scientists, such as Theodore Friedmann, chair of WADA's Gene and Cell Doping Expert Group, raise concerns about the safety of the technology. In another issue of *Play True*, the official publication of WADA, we read:

This technology is highly experimental and completely inappropriate where the goal might be something other than the cure of life-threatening disease like cancer, neurological degenerations and so on. To apply this very immature technology to athletes or to any young, healthy people for the purpose of increasing some already-normal function, in my mind, is unethical and constitutes deliberate professional malpractice.

(WADA 2007, 13)

However, concerns for the safety of the athlete do not automatically constitute sufficient grounds to prohibit individuals from pursuing risks that they voluntarily assume. This for example is the line of argument that Sailors (2015) and Corlett (2014) have aimed at the National Football League in the US in the wake of the recent scandals regarding head injuries and concussions, and the apparent complicity of franchises in the harming of their athlete employees. Much will depend on the confidence and the certainty of the nascent brain science research, but also on ethical analyses of the risk–benefit ratios applying to particular athletes (Lopez Frias and McNamee 2017), and on a proper consideration of the role that the activity plays in the life of the individuals (and closely related others) who assume the risk (Breivik 2007; Olivier 2006). The default position in Western liberal democracies is, after John Stuart Mill, that an individual's moral imperative is to maximise well-being. In such a society individuals are left to pursue the kinds of lives they wish, accepting the kind of risks that they want.

While this way of maximising well-being raises questions in a much broader debate, we are concerned here with genetic engineering and doping. Of the three criteria used to determine candidacy for WADA's Prohibited List of doping methods and substances, it seems that the potential for performance enhancement is a realistic possibility; that potential harm to health is foreseeable, though its likelihood is uncertain; and a case can certainly be made for (though foreseeably also against) the contrary-to-spirit-of-sport criterion.

Without anticipating too much of the ground covered in the next chapter, it is worth questioning one aspect of the spirit-of-sport criterion regarding the fair/unfair distinction. Thus, we might ask when a performance advantage provided by a biological occurring variation, or by an external biotechnological intervention, is to be considered unfair. Analyses of the conceptual dyad fair/unfair advantage as it relates to sports competition are somewhat rare in the philosophy of sport literature, although they have extensive applications beyond the context of this debate, as we discuss in Chapter 8 in relation to hyperandrogenism in female athletes, and in Chapter 9 in the context of the discussion of advantages provided by prosthesis for Paralympic athletes wishing to compete in able-bodied categories.

One philosopher of sport who recently embarked upon an analysis of the concept of advantage is Hämäläinen, who states that 'It is often implicitly assumed that the concept of advantage is unambiguous and unproblematic; only the parameters of fairness pose a challenge. This seems to be an unwarranted assumption' (Hämäläinen 2012, 310). He distinguishes between two kinds of 'advantage' in competition:

'performance' and 'property' advantage. The former is a relationship of superiority between performance numbers possessed by different athletes (or teams) and is defined as follows: 'A has a final performance advantage over B if A has a better final performance number than B.' Examples of performance numbers are the number of seconds that an athlete runs a sprint in, or the numerical score that is the result of a football match. The latter is defined as 'A has an advantage over B in property X if A has a more favourable amount of this property X than B does', where properties are 'constituent parts of competitors and competition environment' (ibid.).

One of the examples of property advantages offered by Hämäläinen is the oxygen carrying property possessed by Finnish cross-country skier Mäntyranta, who won two gold medals in cross-country skiing at the 1964 Winter Olympics in Innsbruck. It was later determined that Mäntyranta had primary familial and congenital polycythemia, a rare genetic mutation characterised by an elevated absolute red blood cell mass and a consequent increase of 25–50% in his blood oxygen carrying capacity (Thompson 2012). Due to his genetic inheritance, Mäntyranta had a property advantage against fellow competitors, i.e. a greater oxygen carrying capacity. It is plausible to speculate that on at least two occasions (the two gold medals won at the Winter Olympics in Innsbruck 1964) this property advantage contributed directly to his performance advantage (the number of minutes or seconds he was able to complete his race in). Note, however, that a property advantage alone does not result in a performance advantage, as other factors contribute to excellence in competition. As remarked above, it is difficult to justifiably reduce something as complex as athletic excellence to a single factor, whether it be anatomical, biological, physiological or psychological. Of course journalists and media commentators often like to single out a certain trait or attribute, but this is not credible. This is why Mäntyranta's property advantage was not deemed to be unfair, as many other property advantages (Eynon et al. 2013) in terms of genetic variations also are not deemed to be unfair.

Cases like Mäntyranta's are not as rare among elite athletes as one might think, or like to think. Endurance athletes in particular have been shown to have mitochondrial variations that increase aerobic capacity and endurance (Ostrander et al. 2009). Acromegaly, a hormonal condition resulting in large hands and feet (and possibly other co-morbidities), is especially prevalent among basketball players (Clemmons 2008). There has also been speculation that Michael Phelps, winner of eight gold medals at the 2008 Beijing Summer Olympics, has Marfan syndrome, a rare genetic condition affecting connective tissues that results in long limbs and flexible joints – an obvious advantage for a swimmer (Doyle 2008). Another example – this time not merely speculative – was Flo Hyman, one of the greatest protagonists of women's volleyball in the 1980s, who was diagnosed post-mortem with Marfan syndrome. The condition gave her tall stature and long arms, obviously an advantage in volleyball (Bostwick and Joyner 2012). As we have noted, what may be a positive abnormality in one context may be debilitating in another: Marfan syndrome was the cause of Hyman's death during a match in 1986 due to aortic dissection.

Mutations that confer an increased muscle bulk in children have been identified at the level of the myostatin gene (Schuelke et al. 2004). While drugs that target the myostatin gene, and gene transfer technologies that mimic the naturally occurring mutations, are included in the WADA Prohibited List, the naturally occurring mutations are represented by the regulators and the media as a source of excellence, and children born with such mutations are encouraged to pursue a career in sport, as depicted in the TV documentary *Extraordinary People* aired in 2011.[12]

All the examples above, and many others, show that elite athletes derive advantages from a range of biological variations, which are cherished and nurtured (with genetic testing and screening programmes, among other more traditional talent identification programmes). As Claire Sullivan points out,

> The fact is the playing field [in elite sports] has never been level. There will always be genetic variations that provide a competitive edge for some athletes over others. We readily accept the genetic, athletic gifts that elite athletes possess without trying to find ways to 'level the playing field'.
>
> *(Sullivan 2011)*

This is because the exceptional biological and genetic variations are considered part of what the elite athlete is, and of what makes sports competitions valuable, namely achieving excellence through combination of talent – the natural endowment of the athlete – and dedicated commitment – the effort in training and preparation that the athlete puts forth to maximise what her talent offers. And of course, there are also systemic biases (Loland 2002) but these are the object of more readily malleable regulation. Nevertheless, all the biological and genetic variations found in elite athletes are deemed ethically acceptable because it is part of the meaning of elite sports to see individuals with exceptional physical characteristics pushing their bodies to the limit to win in competitions and, perhaps, achieving world records. We proceed now to unpack in Chapter 6 what the meaning of sport, or in other words, the spirit of sport, might be, before ethically evaluating in detail in Chapter 7 one real-world example of a gene transfer technology with potentially enhancing effects.

Notes

All websites accessed October 2017.

1 Sections of this chapter were previously published in Camporesi, S. (2014). *From Bench to Bedside, to Track & Field: The Context of Enhancement and its Ethical Relevance*. San Francisco, CA: University of California Medical Humanities Press. ISBN: 978-0-9889865-4-1 (pp. 67–80). We would like to acknowledge Professor Brian Dolan, Editor of UC Medical Humanities Press, for granting us permission to use the content in this volume.

2 http://bioviva-science.com/2016/04/21/first-gene-therapy-successful-against-human-aging

3 The discussion of whether ageing should count as a disease in the first place is beyond the scope of this chapter, but can evidently be linked back to the discussion of the goals of medicine and sport medicine presented in the next chapter.

4 www.wada-ama.org/en/gene-doping-expert-group
5 www.wada-ama.org/en/Science-Medicine/Science-topics/Gene-Doping/
6 www.wada-ama.org/en/gene-doping-expert-group. The full list of up-to-date WADA funded research projects can be found at www.wada-ama.org/en/funded-research-projects
7 One of the authors, Camporesi, worked in this lab in 2006 and 2007.
8 www.kcl.ac.uk/newsevents/news/newsrecords/2012/01Jan/London-2012-unveil-Anti-Doping-Laboratory.aspx
9 www.telegraph.co.uk/sport/olympics/7981501/London-2012-Olympics-Wada-hails-drug-breakthrough-to-combat-cheats.html
10 At proofs stage, we became aware that WADA is adding CRISPR gene-editing agents to its list of banned substances for use in sports. Beginning next year, WADA is to prohibit the use 'gene-editing agents designed to alter genome sequences and/or the transcriptional or epigenetic regulation of gene expression'; www.engadget.com/2017/10/10/wada-banning-sports-gene-editing-doping/
11 http://edition.cnn.com/2009/WORLD/asiapcf/08/03/china.dna.children.ability/
12 www.imdb.com/title/tt1899850/

References

All websites accessed October 2017.

Agar, N. 2008. *Liberal Eugenics: In Defence of Human Enhancement*. New York: John Wiley & Sons.

Aquino Neto, F.R.D., V.F. Sarderla, L. Mirotti and L. Pizzatti. 2016. Running ahead of doping: analytical advances and challenges faced by modern laboratories ahead of Rio 2016. *Bioanalysis*, 8(17): 1753–1756.

Baoutina, A., I.E. Alexander, J.E. Rasko and K.R. Emslie. 2008. Developing strategies for detection of gene doping. *The Journal of Gene Medicine*, 10(1): 3–20.

Baoutina, A., T. Coldham, G.S. Bains and K.R. Emslie. 2010. Gene doping detection: Evaluation of approach for direct detection of gene transfer using erythropoietin as a model system. *Gene Therapy*, 17(8): 1022–1032.

Bartlett, J. 2003. Mighty mice hold hope for muscle ailments. *Penn Current*. Available at: https://penncurrent.upenn.edu/2003-12-11/research/mighty-mice-hold-hope-muscle-ailments

Barton-Davis, E.R., D.I. Shoturma, A. Musaro, N. Rosenthal and H.L. Sweeney. 1998. Viral mediated expression of insulin-like growth factor I blocks the aging-related loss of skeletal muscle function. *Proceedings of the National Academy of Sciences*, 95(26): 15603–15607.

Baumann, G.P. 2012. Growth hormone doping in sports: a critical review of use and detection strategies. *Endocrine Reviews*, 33(2): 155–186.

Borrione, P., A. Mastrone, R.A. Salvo, A. Spaccamiglio, L. Grasso and A. Angeli. 2008. Oxygen delivery enhancers: past, present, and future. *Journal of Endocrinological Investigation*, 31(2): 185–192.

Bostwick, J.M. and M.J. Joyner. 2012. The limits of acceptable biological variation in elite athletes: should sex ambiguity be treated differently from other advantageous genetic traits? *Mayo Clinic Proceedings*, 87(6): 508–513.

Breivik, G. 2007. Can BASE jumping be morally defended? In *Philosophy, Risk and Adventure Sports*, ed. M.J. McNamee. Abingdon: Routledge, pp. 168–185.

Brzeziańska, E., D. Domańska and A. Jegier. 2014. Gene doping in sport – perspectives and risks. *Biology of Sport*, 31(4): 251–259. doi:10.5604/20831862.1120931

Business Standard. 2013. WADA optimistic about gene-doping detection research. Available at: www.business-standard.com/article/news-ians/wada-optimistic-about-gene-doping-detection-research-113060700336_1.html

Campisi, J. and F.D.A. di Fagagna. 2007. Cellular senescence: when bad things happen to good cells. *Nature Reviews. Molecular Cell Biology*, 8(9): 729–740.

Camporesi, S. 2017. An alternative solution to lifting the ban on doping: breaking the payoff matrix of professional sport by shifting liability away from athletes. *Sport, Ethics and Philosophy*, 11(1): 109–118.

Camporesi, S. and M.J. McNamee. 2014. Performance enhancement, elite athletes and anti doping governance: comparing human guinea pigs in pharmaceutical research and professional sports. *Philosophy, Ethics, and Humanities in Medicine*, 9(1), 4.

Clemmons, A.K. 2008. 7 feet 7 and 360 pounds, with bigger feet than Shaq's. *The New York Times*, 9 January. Available at: www.nytimes.com/2008/01/09/sports/ncaabasketball/09a sheville.html?_r=0

Corlett, J.A. 2014. Should inter-collegiate football be eliminated? Assessing the arguments philosophically. *Sport, Ethics and Philosophy*, 8(2): 116–136.

Devine, J.W. 2010. Doping is a threat to sporting excellence. *British Journal of Sports Medicine*, 45: 637–639.

Dimeo, P., T.M. Hunt and R. Horbury. 2011. The individual and the state: a social historical analysis of the East German 'doping system'. *Sport in History*, 31(2): 218–237.

Doyle, J. 2008. Michael Phelps unintentionally raises Marfan Syndrome awareness. *Fox News*, 21 August. Available at: www.foxnews.com/story/2008/08/21/michael-phelps-unin tentionally-raises-marfan-syndrome-awareness.html

Eynon, N., E.D. Hanson, A. Lucia, P.J. Houweling, F. Garton, K.N. North and D.J. Bishop. 2013. Genes for elite power and sprint performance: ACTN3 leads the way. *Sports Medicine*, 43(9): 803–817.

Fantz, A. 2010. The new frontier in athletic doping – genes. *CNN*. Available at: http://edition.cnn.com/2010/HEALTH/02/19/genetic.doping/index.html

Fischetto, G. and S. Bermon. 2013. From gene engineering to gene modulation and manipulation: can we prevent or detect gene doping in sports? *Sports Medicine*, 43(10): 965–977.

Foddy, B. and J. Savulescu. 2007. Ethics of performance enhancement in sport: drugs and gene doping. In *Principles of Health Care Ethics*, 2nd edn, eds R. Ashcroft, A. Dawson et al. Chichester, UK: Wiley, pp. 511–519.

Franke, W.W. and B. Berendonk. 1997. Hormonal doping and androgenization of athletes: a secret program of the German Democratic Republic government. *Clinical Chemistry*, 43 (7): 1262–1279.

Giacca, M. and S. Zacchigna. 2012. Virus-mediated gene delivery for human gene therapy. *Journal of Controlled Release*, 161(2): 377–388.

Haisma, H.J. and O. De Hon. 2006. Gene doping. *International Journal of Sports Medicine*, 27 (04): 257–266.

Hämäläinen, M. 2012. The concept of advantage in sport. *Sport, Ethics and Philosophy*, 6(3): 308–322.

Harridge, S.D. and C.P. Velloso. 2008. Gene doping. *Essays in Biochemistry*, 44: 125–138.

Harris, E. 2009. Eight scientists who became their own guinea pigs. *New Scientist*, 11 March. Available at: www.newscientist.com/article/dn16735-eight-scientists-who-became-their-own-guinea-pigs/

Hoberman, J.M. 2001. *Mortal Engines: The Science of Performance and the Dehumanization of Sport*. Caldwell, NJ: Blackburn Press.

Hollon, T. 2000. Researchers and regulators reflect on first gene therapy death. *Nature Medicine*, 6(1): 6–7.

Jager, L. and A. Ehrhardt. 2007. Emerging adenoviral vectors for stable correction of genetic disorders. *Current Gene Therapy*, 74: 272–283.

Lehrman, S. 1999. Virus treatment questioned after gene therapy death. *Nature*, 401: 517–518.

Le Page, M. 2016. Gene doping in sport could make the Olympics fairer and safer. *New Scientist*, 5 August. Available at: www.newscientist.com/article/2100181-gene-doping-in-sport-could-make-the-olympics-fairer-and-safer/

Leuenberger, N., C. Reichel and F. Lasne. 2012. Detection of erythropoiesis-stimulating agents in human anti-doping control: past, present and future. *Bioanalysis*, 4(13): 1565–1575.

Li, Z., B. Zhao, Y.S. Kim, C.Y. Hu and J. Yang. 2010. Administration of a mutated myostatin propeptide to neonatal mice significantly enhances skeletal muscle growth. *Molecular Reproduction and Development*, 77(1): 76–82.

Loland, S. 2002. Technology in sport: three ideal-typical views and their implications. *European Journal of Sport Science*, 2(1): 1–11.

Loland, S. 2017. Education in anti-doping: the art of self-imposed constraints. In *Acute Topics in Anti-Doping*, eds O. Rabin and Y. Pitsiladis. Basel: Karger Publishers, pp. 153–159.

Lopez Frias, F.J. and M. McNamee. 2017. Ethics, brain injuries, and sports: prohibition, reform, and prudence. *Sport, Ethics and Philosophy*, 11(3): 264–280.

McFarlane, C., G.Z. Hui, W.Z.W. Amanda, H.Y. Lau, S. Lokireddy, G. XiaoJia ... and R. Kambadur. 2011. Human myostatin negatively regulates human myoblast growth and differentiation. *American Journal of Physiology-Cell Physiology*, 301(1): C195–C203.

Macedo, A., M. Moriggi, M. Vasso, S. De Palma, M. Sturnega, G. Friso ... and S. Zacchigna. 2011. Enhanced athletic performance on multisite AAV-IGF1 gene transfer coincides with massive modification of the muscle proteome. *Human Gene Therapy*, 23(2): 146–157.

Miah, A. 2004. *Genetically Modified Athletes: Biomedical Ethics, Gene Doping and Sport*. London: Routledge.

Murray, Y. 2009. Ethics and endurance enhancing technologies in sport. In *Performance-enhancing Technologies in Sports: Ethical, Conceptual, and Scientific Issues*, eds T.H. Murray, K.J. Maschke and A.A. Wasunna. Baltimore: John Hopkins University Press, pp. 115–124.

Naish, J. 2012. Genetically modified athletes: forget drugs. *Daily Mail*, 1 August. Available at: www.dailymail.co.uk/news/article-2181873/Genetically-modified-athletes-Forget-drugs-There-suggestions-Chinese-athletes-genes-altered-make-stronger.html

Olivier, S. 2006. Moral dilemmas of participation in dangerous leisure activities. *Leisure Studies*, 25(1): 95–109.

Østergård, T., J. Ek, Y. Hamid, B. Saltin, O.B. Pedersen, T. Hansen and O. Schmitz. 2005. Influence of the PPAR-γ2 Pro12Ala and ACE I/D polymorphisms on insulin sensitivity and training effects in healthy offspring of type 2 diabetic subjects. *Hormone and Metabolic research*, 37(02): 99–105.

Ostrander, E.A., H.J. Huson and G.K. Ostrander. 2009. Genetics of athletic performance. *Annual Review of Genomics and Human Genetics*, 10: 407–429.

Polcz, S. and A. Lewis. 2016. CRISPR-Cas9 and the non-germline non-controversy. *Journal of Law and Biosciences*, January 2016. doi:10.2139/ssrn.2697333

Regalado, A. 2015. A tale of do-it-yourself gene therapy. *MIT Technology Review*, 14 October. Available at: www.technologyreview.com/s/542371/a-tale-of-do-it-yourself-gene-therapy/

Reichel, C. 2011. OMICS-strategies and methods in the fight against doping. *Forensic Science International*, 213(1): 20–34.

Reynolds, G. 2007. Outlaw DNA. *New York Times*, 3 June. Available at: www.nytimes.com/2007/06/03/sports/playmagazine/0603play-hot.html

Rupert, J.L. 2009. Transcriptional profiling: a potential anti-doping strategy. *Scandinavian Journal of Medicine & Science in Sports*, 19(6): 753–763.

Sailors, P.R. 2015. Personal foul: an evaluation of the moral status of football. *Journal of the Philosophy of Sport*, 42(2): 269–286.

Schneider, A.J. and T. Friedmann. 2006. Gene transfer in sports: an opening scenario for genetic enhancement of normal 'human traits'. *Advances in Genetics*, 51: 37–49.

Schuelke, M., K.R. Wagner, L.E. Stolz, C. Hübner, T. Riebel, W. Kömen and S.J. Lee. 2004. Myostatin mutation associated with gross muscle hypertrophy in a child. *New England Journal of Medicine*, 350(26): 2682–2688.

Shawi, M. and C. Autexier. 2008. Telomerase, senescence and ageing. *Mechanisms of Ageing and Development*, 129(1): 3–10.

Sullivan, C.F. 2011. Gender verification and gender policies in elite sport: eligibility and 'fair play'. *Journal of Sport and Social Issues*, 35(4): 400–419.

Thompson, H. 2012. Superhuman athletes. *Nature*, 487(7407): 287–289.

Ungerleider, S. 2001. *Faust's Gold: Inside the East German Doping Machine*. London: Macmillan.

Vlahovich, N., P.A. Fricker, M.A. Brown and D. Hughes. 2016. Ethics of genetic testing and research in sport: a position statement from the Australian Institute of Sport. *British Journal of Sports Medicine*: 1–7.

WADA. 2007. *Play True*, issue 2: *Science: Honing in on Doping*. Available at: www.wada-ama. org/sites/default/files/resources/files/PlayTrue_2007_2_Science_Honing_In_On_Doping_ EN.pdf

WADA. 2008. *Play True*, issue 3: *Levelling the Playing Field*. Available at: www.wada-ama.org/ sites/default/files/resources/files/PlayTrue_2008_3_Levelling_the_Playing_Field_EN.pdf

WADA. 2015. *World Anti-doping Code*. Available at: www.wada-ama.org/en/what-we-do/ the-code

WADA. 2017. *List of Prohibited Substances and Methods*. Available at: www.wada-ama.org/ en/prohibited-list

Warmflash, D. 2016. Should we trust experiments on one patient? Lessons from BioViva's anti-aging gene therapy. *Genetic Literacy Project*, 10 May. Available at: https://geneticlitera cyproject.org/2016/05/10/trust-experiments-one-patient-lessons-biovivas-anti-aging-gene-therapy/

Wells, D.J. 2008. Gene doping: the hype and the reality. *British Journal of Pharmacology*, 154(3): 623–631.

Zentilin, L., U. Puligadda, V. Lionetti, S. Zacchigna, C. Collesi, L. Pattarini ... and F.A. Recchia. 2010. Cardiomyocyte VEGFR-1 activation by VEGF-B induces compensatory hypertrophy and preserves cardiac function after myocardial infarction. *The FASEB Journal*, 24(5): 1467–1478.

PART II

Enhancement, Therapy, and the Ethical Construction of Categories in Sport

6

ENHANCEMENT, DOPING AND THE SPIRIT OF SPORT

6.1 Introduction[1]

John Hoberman was among the first to discuss bioethical issues in the contexts of high-performance sport, and to realise that human nature, and what it means to be human, are at stake in discussions of what directions professional sport will take (Hoberman 1992). One important context for his reflections was the East German sports medicine/sports science nexus which saw a country with only 16 million inhabitants ranked second in track and field according to Olympic gold medals won in the 1976 and 1980 Olympic Games. Clearly, the combination of political ideology and medical science has notorious forebears, but this was a remarkable feat. Nevertheless, the costs of such success were to be revealed somewhat later. One of the athletes, the former women's world sprint relay record holder Ines Geipel, referred to her experiences as 'a large experiment, a big chemical field test'.[2] German heptathlete Birgit Dressel is another example (cf. Camporesi and McNamee 2014). Birgit Dressel was born in Bremen, West Germany, in 1960. She came in ninth at the 1984 Olympic Games in Los Angeles, and fourth at the 1986 European Championships in Stuttgart, West Germany. She died on 10 April 1987 due to multiple organ failure caused by the combination of pharmaceuticals she had been ingesting over the past months aiming to enhance her athletic performance. In response to her mother's anxieties, Dressel is reported to have said 'These are all harmless drugs. All athletes take them. It's really nothing special' (*Time Magazine* 1988). An autopsy revealed traces of 101 different medications in her body, including bovine tissue (Harvey 1988). The investigation report on her death concluded that despite her powerful appearance Birgit Dressel was the opposite of a healthy person: as reported in the German newspaper *Der Spiegel*, Dressel was 'in truth a chronically sick young woman pumped full with hundreds of drugs. Sport had made a cripple of her long ago, destroying her joints and ruining her internal organs prematurely' (*Der Spiegel* 1987).

Looking back on that period Hoberman summarises, perhaps a little rhetorically, that 'The bioethical crisis of sport is a crisis of human engineering in which our concept of human nature itself is at stake' (Hoberman 1992, 32). He is not alone in that view. It is not coincidental that the US President's Report of 2003, commissioned to explore the moral limits of biotechnology, pondered on the future of human nature, in part via the lens of sports. Chair of the US Council on Bioethics at that time, the self-confessed 'bioconservative' Leon Kass, wrote that 'human nature itself lies on the operating table, ready for alteration, for eugenic and neuropsychic "enhancement", for wholesale design' (Kass 2003, 4).

Given the central role of medical research in driving developments in pharmacology and genetics, and the subsequent application of therapies to the quest for the enhancement of athlete performance, the therapy/enhancement distinction has assumed a hugely significant role in bioethical scholarship over the last 20 years. It has also played a significant role in the scholarship of doping in athletics, both of a genetic and non-genetic kind. In this chapter we critically present some of these debates in the contexts of the emerging field of sports medicine ethics (McNamee 2016) in order to shed light on the ethics of genetic engineering and doping.

6.2 The emergence of the athletic body as an 'abnormal' entity and the goals of sport medicine

The coalescence of sports and medicine is doubtless a relationship that goes back to antiquity (Berryman and Park 1992; Leadbetter and Leadbetter 1996). During the growth of modern sport the physical differences between population norms and elite athletes was not so marked, yet as the twentieth century proceeded the notion of elite athlete became constructed as a distinct category or class of individual (Heggie 2011). The emerging specialisation of sport training and support, along with population-wide changes in human nutrition, growth and development, generated athletes who were bigger, faster and stronger. As sport has become highly commercialised it has also become heavily medicalised over the course of the twentieth and twenty-first centuries, and the question of normality for the elite athlete has also changed. Heggie notes how at the beginning of the twentieth century 'the definition of the normal athlete essentially overlapped with that of the normal, healthy citizen' (ibid., 4). However, over the following years, 'these categories were gradually separated, as the athletic body began to be medically, scientifically and socially constructed as a discrete physiological or clinical entity' (ibid.). By the 1950s, elite athletes were constructed as a separate category different from the 'rest of us'.

In organisational terms, the specialism is a twentieth-century innovation. The Fédération Internationale de Médecine Sportive (FIMS) was established in 1928, and the first book to use the title 'sports medicine' appeared in the 1930s: Dr Herbert Herxheimer's *Grundriss der Sportmedizin* (Foundations of Sports Medicine) (Carter 2013). Despite these precursors, the founding of the American College of Sports Medicine, by physical educators and physicians, only occurred in 1954, and it was not until 2005 that the specialism was officially recognised in British medi-cine.[3] The collection of social and economic processes that generate a medical specialism are many and varied. In his early classic on sports injuries, Williams (1962, 265–316) had argued that there is no such thing as a *sui generis* category of sport injury – rather there are simply injuries that arise in the contexts of sports. Under this conception we simply have medicine, largely orthopaedics, applied to sports populations. By contrast, Heggie (2011, 17) argues that the genesis of the specialism is predicated on a 'clinically distinct patient group', one that is abnormal in a pathological or enhanced manner. In order to examine the nature and goals of sports medicine it is necessary to consider the goals of medicine more broadly, and then to consider the role that the therapy/enhancement distinction may play in it.

Modern discussion of the goals of medicine in the bioethics literature has its roots in a 1996 report commissioned by the Hastings Center, which was the result of an international task force including medical doctors and ethicists from the US, the UK, several countries in mainland Europe, South America, China and Indonesia. What prompted the task force at that time was the need to inform the discussion on how biomedical advances should impact on the decisions about the allocation of scarce resources in healthcare (Allert et al. 1996).

The report outlined four key goals for medicine:

1.   Prevention of disease and injury, and promotion and maintenance of health;
2.   Relief of pain and suffering caused by maladies;
3.   Care and cure of those with a malady, and the care of those who cannot be cured;
4.   Avoidance of premature death and the pursuit of a peaceful death.

Underlying all four goals is the principle that 'medicine cannot have as a goal the ultimate well-being, beyond the aim of good health, of the individual'. It is clear that the account of medicine here is essentially a therapeutic one, in which enhancements, whatever they are taken to mean, seem to have no role to play. There is much, however, to argue with in this account. The notion of health is a deeply contested concept. Accounts range from allegedly value-free accounts to those that incorporate subjective elements at their heart. Thus, while all commen-tators might agree that some version of goal 1 is an essential goal of medicine, its precise specification is open to very wide interpretation. Similarly, consider the second part of the first goal: what counts as 'promotion' of health? It depends on what is understood as health, and what are the limits of its 'promotion'. Moreover, with respect to goal 4 it is far from clear what would constitute a premature death. Ought the reference class to be simply determined by a statistically derived number of years, or might it be limited to a Western narrative regarding the achievement of certain goals in life, such as the standard middle-class goals of achieving a career, having a family, owning a house, seeing the children go to college, getting married and starting to build their own families? Or might it be something quite different?

This alerts us to the fact that the central concepts in the discussion, such as what counts as 'prevention' of disease and injury and 'promotion' of health, are value-laden. If we now have a technology (say, CRISPR genome editing) through which we might be able to screen out all kinds of genetic diseases by editing the human embryos, should we do so? Would that count as an instance of medical intervention proper? (cf. Scully and Rehmann-Sutter 2001)

Further, we must ask what follows if these four goals are also thought to be definitive in relation to sports medicine. Two things might first strike us. First if we consider these to be the goals of sports medicine *because* they are the goals of all medicine, then we have a therapeutic approach to sports medicine (treatment, prevention *qua* health promotion), where any claim to the uniqueness or distinctness of sports medicine seems to fall flat (cf. Johnson 2004; Green 2004). Moreover, what seems to distinguish it as an independent branch of medicine, namely the goal of enhancing athletes' capacities, appears beyond the scope of medicine itself (Edwards and McNamee 2006).

This restrictive reading of sports medicine and its ethical basis seem to be in tension with a recent commentary on the ethics of prescribing neurological enhancements for the American Medical Association Journal of Medicine, which concludes that although physicians are not morally obliged (i.e. do not have a moral duty) to prescribe neurological enhancements (and may refuse to do so if they consider the prescription to fall outside the goals of their profession), they may do so. In other words, the prescription of a drug with clear enhancement purposes, although not being morally obligatory, is morally permissible. This view is encapsulated in the recent American Academy of Neurology (AAN) guidelines. It seems that the AAN is drawing a distinction between what is ethically required and what is ethically permissible, leaving the decision to the individual practitioner (Larriviere et al. 2009). What this entails in practice, though, is that, at least in the US, patients could go 'doctor-shopping' until they find a suitable doctor for their needs.

According to Hoberman (2014), we are seeing the exportation of the norms of sports medicine (enhancement) more broadly into medicine. He has forcefully argued that 'physician-assisted doping' has transformed high-performance sport into a 'chronically overmedicated subculture'. He writes: 'The doping doctors of the sports world have pioneered "entrepreneurial" medical practices that are now available to enormous numbers of people in search of hormonal rejuvenation' (ibid., 572). Yet his representation of the doping doctors of sport is at least partially historically inaccurate, since the prescription of testosterone for anti-ageing or to increase sexual performance is not a recent evolution. As a matter of fact, testosterone has been prescribed in the US to increase sexual performance for at least the past 100 years, as narrated by American historians of medicine Rothman and Rothman in their book *The Pursuit of Perfection* (Rothman and Rothman 2003). Already in the early 1900s, the pioneering American surgeon Max Thorek was known for performing 'therapeutical gonadal implantations' with the aim of elevating the level of male hormones and sexual function in older patients.

Between 1912 and 1923, Thorek performed more than a hundred testicular transplants at the American Hospital in Chicago. These were testicular transplants collected mostly from apes and monkeys, but also from human cadavers (ibid., 142–144). Thorek was also one of the first surgeons to perform breast reduction and abdominal excisions (the antecedents of contemporary plastic surgery practices). In 1942, Thorek wrote one of the first textbooks on plastic surgery.

As a physician, Thorek is a particularly interesting foil for our discussion of enhancement and the norms of medicine, as he firmly believed that enhancement interventions lay within the scope of medicine, and his ideas can be seen as fore-runners of some of the arguments used today in support of pharmacological enhancement. For example, he was convinced that 'raising the quotient of patient happiness' was a legitimate medical task, which could be pursued within the purview of the doctor's remit. He wrote: 'If surgery can restore happiness and enjoyment of life to an individual who has lost them, that is as strong a justification for its use as restoration to health' (Rothman and Rothman 2003, 143).

It seems, then, that simply articulating an account of the goals of medicine from which we may deduce some easy priority of one set of interventions (therapeutic) over another (enhancements) is problematic. We turn then to a review of the salient points in the many debates over the therapy/enhancement distinction in order to shed further light on doping in sports.

6.3 The therapy/enhancement distinction at work in medicine and sport medicine

The genesis of the therapy/enhancement distinction is somewhat disputed. Some scholars argue that it arose in the context of the discussion of gene therapy in the US in the late 1980s, with the purpose of demarcating ethically legitimate applications of gene transfer technologies from other questionable applications (Camporesi 2014). At the time of the first gene therapy clinical trials, the use of gene transfer to treat severe immunological diseases was considered morally justifi-able, even though risks for the individuals were very high, because of the severity of the disease (in the case of the early trials, it was adenosine deaminase deficiency, a genetic disease that damages the immune system of the sufferer, seriously depleting their ability to fend off diseases) and of the absence of alternative treatments. However, people were worried about the prospect of other uses of gene transfer techniques, which would put subjects at a high risk without the same justification as the treatment of a life-threatening condition. Others, not wholly disputing the case above, argue that it was driven by the need of medical insurers to determine those conditions for which it would pay for its customers to be treated (Buchanan et al. 2001; Daniels 2000). The distinction thus serves to rein-force the insurers' grip on their policies and thus their profits. Equally, under conditions of scarce resources one could see how managers within a nationally funded system might use the distinction not necessarily drawn at the same points, to maximise the efficiency of their limited resources.

Rather than simply attempting to conceptually analyse and articulate some decisive line to demarcate the two concepts, it seems now to be widely agreed that what is called for is a consideration of the use to which the distinction can be put. A number of scholars have argued that the distinction cannot plausibly be used since all therapies can be seen as enhancements from the individual's perspective (Murray 2009: Holm and McNamee 2011). The oft-cited case of immunisation serves to show how one and the same intervention can be therapeutic for some, but enhancing beyond the normal range for a particular patient, in which case a preventative intervention would count as an enhancement (cf. Harris 2010). And the same might be said *ceteris paribus* for the use of antibiotics or cholesterol lowering drugs. Moreover, as will be noted in the following chapters, the use of human growth hormone may normalise height in a person suffering from dwarfism or indeed may enhance the overall height of a merely small person, as in the case of Lionel Messi, five-time winner of the *ballon d'or*, the highest award for an individual footballer (soccer player).

In the light of these remarks, we can see how one important use of the distinction might be to serve as a professional boundary within medicine, or even a moral one. Therapeutic interventions tied to cure and care and aiming at normal health are to be approved of, while enhancements over and above that norm are neither 'medical' nor admirable. And we can also see why one might advocate a distinction based on something like an understanding of normal functioning in order to bolster the distinction in a context-free way. It provides decision-makers with an apparently decisive answer to practical and policy questions, such as those regarding allocation of services or other resources. One influential bioconservative use of the distinction is at the heart of the report of the (US) President's Council on Bioethics (2003) entitled *Beyond Therapy: Biotechnology and the Pursuit of Happiness*, already mentioned above. The distinction draws upon the most famous account of health as 'normal species functioning' and enhancement as 'beyond species typical functioning'. According to this interpretation, a therapeutic intervention aims at restoring health or, following Boorse (1977), species-typical normal functioning.

Boorse's Biostatistical Theory of health (BST), formed over a series of essays, holds that health is defined as the statistically typical contribution of all the organism's parts and processes to the organism's overall goals of survival and reproduction (Boorse 1977, 1997). He aimed to define health in a value-free, objective, way. Boorse himself does not argue that normative facts flow from such an account, nor could he while arguing for a naturalistic (some might say positivistic) account of health (Kluka 2015). However, from an ontological perspective, as scholars such as Kingma (2007), Scully (2014), Scully and Rehmann-Sutter (2001), Eilers et al. (2014), Mills (2011, 2015) and Schües (2014) have pointed out, no definition of health can ever be value-free: what counts as normal and as healthy is context-dependent and value-laden and, consequently, so is the concept of enhancement. It is in this sense that normal functioning, like normal health, is inescapably normative.

Sometimes what is at stake is the role that human nature itself plays in these debates. While the scientifically minded, such as Boorse (often referred to as naturalists), claim that the facts of human nature entail no ethical or normative power or significance, others like Kass (2003) and Sandel (2004) do. To these and like-minded scholars, biotechnologists who recognise no limits to their interventions are like a modern-day Prometheus. One difficulty for such a claim is that in classical sources there is not one but two renderings of the myth of Prometheus (McNamee 2007). Hesiod's account is a morality tale – beware of human hubris that would defy the gods. Aeschylus underplays Prometheus's disrespect of the gods and celebrates his cunning deceit of them. The point is that genetics, like other forms of medical or biotechnology, challenges our sense of the limits of human beings both in terms of what powers we have and how we understand the limits of the species.

Yet this was not entirely a new warning against the unfettered advances of biotechnology, As Jonas had written 50 years before:

> The biological control of man, especially genetic control, raises ethical questions of a wholly new kind for which neither previous praxis nor previous thought has prepared us. Since no less than the nature and image of man are at issue, prudence itself becomes our first ethical duty, and hypothetical reasoning our first responsibility.
>
> *(Jonas 1974, 141)*

Sandel's position is that perfectionism, i.e. the perfection, or 'optimisation', of human nature, is a notion that must be understood to have normative limits (Sandel 2004). Hence he claims that some forms of genetic modification attempt to obliterate the giftedness of human nature which, for him, is predicated on the notion that our gifts and achievements are to a certain extent 'given', not merely acquired. He points out that this principle admits of both theological and non-theological ethical readings. One working-out of this idea aligns closely with our discussion of children and genetic testing in Chapter 3 of this volume. He writes:

> To appreciate children as gifts is to accept them as they come, not as objects of our design, or products of our will, or instruments of our ambition. Parental love is not contingent on the talents and attributes the child happens to have. ... [We] do not choose our children. Their qualities are unpredictable, and even the most conscientious parents cannot be held wholly responsible for the kind of child they have. That is why parenthood, more than other human relationships, teaches what the theologian William F. May calls an 'openness to the unbidden'.
>
> *(Sandel 2004: 45)*

This objection of the use of biotechnologies to dominate present and future narratives has deep and wide appeal. It is central to our sense of caring guidance of the vulnerability of the child. But does it hold as much weight with competent adults plotting their own scientific or athletic narratives? Sandel sets out a litmus test for our would-be admiration of enhanced and non-enhanced athletes. His criteria of demarcation amount to a virtue-ethical consideration and a naturalistic account of the value of sports: we admire the virtuous perfection of natural talent[4] more than we do mere meritocracy. We may be grudging in our praise for the schoolchild who because of her innate gifts or early maturation beats everyone in the school sportsday sprint. We also admire those less gifted, who simply put in the hard yards of commitment, sacrifice and dedication to improve upon less well-endowed beginnings. Yet ultimately what counts is how one performs, not merely how hard one tries (at least in elite sport). Thus Sandel acknowledges the importance of effort but limits the modes of perfection to those that do not usurp the giftedness athletic talent. Genetic modification would count as a prime example – hence the title of his chapter on sports in *The Case Against Perfection* (Sandel 2004): 'Bionic athletes'. However, those technologies that enhance performances by enabling natural talent to flourish are acceptable.

Bioliberals such as Julian Savulescu and John Harris have pointed to simple examples that provide difficult cases for the distinction, such as interventions to resist tooth decay that few would deny as legitimately medical interventions. More widely, they argue that, as we live longer, old people increasingly die of diseases associated with old age, such that life-extending treatment of diseases associated with old age would count as both therapy and enhancement. Their general position is that the therapy/enhancement distinction is irrelevant from a moral point of view. They argue that both therapy and enhancement should be granted in order to promote individuals' well-being, regardless of statistically imposed measurements and evaluations. Indeed, Harris (2010) goes as far as to say that we have a duty to enhance our children to create better lives for them, no less than we must help them to avoid harmful conditions.

This criticism aligns with sociologists and philosophers who reject an inherently ethical (typically vocational/deontological) formulation of the profession of medicine itself, seeing it as one among many occupations concerned with human well-being. Authors such as the libertarian Engelhardt (1990) hold that medicine has no intrinsically ethical domain or essence, over and above the contract or agreement that exists between the physician and the patient. Neither therapy nor enhancement is afforded any particular ethical status *qua* the physician's intervention. The physician simply responds to the patient's health-related desires, and intervenes according to their conception of what is good for them.

Other critics, whom one could neither label bioconservative nor bioliberal, have objections to the distinction and its appeal to human nature as a basis for normative evaluations such as those regarding the desirability or otherwise of genetic interventions. Lewens not only argues that the distinction cannot play the demarcating role that the authors of the *Beyond Therapy* report wanted it to play; but also that the distinction cannot be drawn at all. However, he adds, this should not worry us, since 'new and interesting' questions arise when the distinction is shown to crumble (Lewens 2015). For example, if we were discussing a particular technology aimed at selecting certain traits in human embryos, the new and interesting question would become which values are worth preserving in each trait under consideration, not whether they fall on one side or the other of the distinction.

Norman Daniels offers a limited defence of the distinction. He argues that although the distinction lacks analytical precision it does tidy up some major intuitions and is aligned to considerable convergence in practice. He writes that it has become a 'focal point for convergence in our public conception of what we owe each other by way of medical assistance or healthcare protection' (Daniels 2000, 318). He concludes that, from a practical point of view, the therapy/ enhancement distinction can play a *prima facie* role in demarcating acceptable uses of the technology which could be considered as 'medical necessity' from uses of the technology that go beyond the concept of 'medical necessity'. This *prima facie* role, though, needs to withstand scrutiny and may not constitute a sufficient reason to treat similar cases in dissimilar ways. Thus, in the case of our short-statured patient, only those children with a genetically identified cause might be permitted to receive growth hormone therapy, while those who are short for other reasons, such as poverty or malnutrition, might not. Yet Daniels argues that differential reimbursement is not justified, and that basing medical allocation decisions only on genetic factors is fundamentally unfair.

Where does this brief coverage of a weighty dispute leave us? It is undeniable that the therapy/enhancement distinction is widely used, whatever its philosophical merits turn out to be. It is clear, as Daniels says, that while there are hard cases that it cannot cope with, it can serve satisfactorily to mark a boundary for various health-related purposes. There is some consensus, however, that it cannot unpro- blematically serve to mark a clear ethical boundary between the obligatory and the merely desirable, or the admirable versus the suspect. In this regard, his position may be seen as a working-out of one of Aristotle's most famous dictums. At the beginning of the *Nichomachean Ethics* Aristotle writes:

> It is a mark of the trained mind never to expect more precision in the treat- ment of any subject than the nature of that subject permits; for demanding logical demonstrations from a teacher of rhetoric is clearly about as reasonable as expecting mere plausibility from a mathematician.
>
> *(Barnes et al. 1976, book 1: 3, 116–121)*

If we are ethically to evaluate the ethics of enhancement on a case by case basis (cf. Camporesi 2014) we must ask how much precision we might expect from the therapy/enhancement distinction in the contexts of sports. More specifically, we will pursue the question of what legitimate employment it might have in the discussions of doping and of genetic enhancements in the context of the global regulatory framework: the World Anti-Doping Code (WADC).

6.4 Emergence of anti-doping regulations

It is not easy to determine precisely when and where the idea that doping violates the spirit of sport came into existence. Ritchie (2014) presents a careful historical tracing of the concept in his discussion of Baron Pierre de Coubertin's construction of the concept of Olympism, while Gleaves and Llewellyn (2014) trace the cultural roots of anti-doping to early twentieth-century debates over amateurism. Ritchie cites the influence of Lord Porritt, the New Zealand sprinter-cum-doctor who came third in the famous 'Chariots of Fire' Olympic sprint final in Paris. Porritt was a key force in the establishment of sports medicine, and derided the character of the 'dope' as a kind of moral recalcitrant. Both Dimeo (2007) and Ritchie (2014) unpack some of the ideological content of the early development of anti-doping policy (ADP), which served both to preserve the alleged purity of sport and to sustain its tarnished amateur ideals.

Ideology aside, sport has long been an arena where performance enhancement has been heavily regulated. Unsurprisingly, then, it has thus served as a testing ground for enhancement technologies, for anti-enhancement regulation and for testing public reaction to genetic and other enhancements. Contrary to what may be thought, the administration of substances with the aim to enhance athletic performance has not always been viewed negatively. For a long time, what we now consider 'doping' was viewed as a unremarkable way to extend the athlete's capabilities, and sport was seen as the experimental terrain *par excellence* where it was possible to do so. Trying to enhance one's own athletic performance with any available means was understood as the natural human reaction to coping with fatigue, and competition in sports was first understood as a challenge between athletes and fatigue, and only secondly between athletes and their competitors.

In this sense, the professional athlete was using his own body as the subject of experimentation, and the athlete himself (such was the gendered nature of sport at the time the male designation is warranted) became an experimental subject. This identification of the athlete's body with an experimental terrain can be dated back to 1894, when the pioneering French sports physician Philippe Tissié began to administer several types of beverages to cyclists to test their value as performance enhancers. In this sense, Tissié regarded the elite athlete as an experimental subject whose exertions and trauma could shed light on as yet unexplained human physiology, in a kind of reverse extrapolation from the track and field to the bedside (Hoberman 1992).

Sportive nationalism was another driver for the emergence of this idea, as in the first decade of the twentieth century scientists were accusing each other across the Atlantic to hide the possession of a supposedly secret formula to combat fatigue (Hoberman 1992). In the beginning, objections of 'reprehensible doping' focused more on the medical dangers for the athlete's health (a form of paternalism which is still present in WADA's Prohibited List) than on the idea that doping was a form of cheating which would violate the spirit of sport, as it is now understood. That idea of sportsmanship as fair play emerged in parallel to the commercialisation of sports and its increasing importance as mass culture in the 1920s and 1930s. By the 1950s, Sir Adolphe Abrahams, an honorary medical officer to the International Athletics Board and the British Olympic team, had begun to articulate the difficulties of distinguishing between legitimate and less legitimate means to enhance athletic performance. He wrote that although 'We have to attempt to draw a line where legitimate measures end and reprehensible practices begin' (Abrahams 1958, 26), drawing such a line was not easy at all, and the distinction remained largely a matter of opinion and of conscience.

The International Olympic Committee (IOC) established its first list of banned substances in 1967 as a response to the death of the cyclist Knud Erik Jensen, which was believed to be causally linked to substance misuse – a point whose veracity is challenged by some historians of sport (Møller 2005). Decades of doping, reaching its zenith in the East German system, proceeded in sports across the board. Even after the Ben Johnson/Charlie Francis scandals of the 1988 Seoul Olympics, and the subsequent Dubin enquiry, international federations and the Olympic movement seemed to turn a blind eye to manifest doping across a broad range of sports. Then, in 1999, partly as a reaction to the widespread Tour de France doping scandals of 1998, the IOC convened the first World Conference on Doping in Sport. This event led to the creation on 10 November 1999 of the World Anti-Doping Agency (WADA), with the explicit aim of harmonising anti-doping policies and measures worldwide. WADA is based on cooperation between sports organisations and governments, and is financed by both on an equal basis. Harmonisation relates not only to testing controls and protocols, but also to the development of systems that permit location, identification and monitoring of elite athletes. Nearly all international sports federations have accepted the WADC, and governments support WADA financially (McNamee and Tarasti 2010).

The fundamental rationale for the World Anti-Doping Code is outlined at the beginning of the code, where we can read:

> Anti-doping programs seek to preserve what is intrinsically valuable about sport. This intrinsic value is often referred to as '*the spirit of sport*' [italics ours]. It is the essence of Olympism, the pursuit of human excellence through the dedicated perfection of each person's natural talents. It is how we play true. The spirit of sport is the celebration of the human spirit, body and mind, and is reflected in values we find in and through sport, including:
> • Ethics, fair play and honesty • Health • Excellence in performance • Character and education • Fun and joy • Teamwork • Dedication and commitment • Respect for rules and laws • Respect for self and other Participants • Courage • Community and solidarity. Doping is fundamentally contrary to the spirit of sport.[5]

McNamee (2012, 2016) has noted, contrary to some sweeping criticisms of WADA raised by others (Foddy and Savulescu 2007; Savulescu 2016), how the apparent simplicity of the process of inclusion of a substance in WADA's Pro-hibited List is deceptive. Article 1 sets out the definition of doping. Doping does not consist simply of the ingestion of a prohibited substance, but is rather defined procedurally, which means that doping is defined as the occurrence of one or more of the anti-doping rule violations (ADRVs) set forth from Article 2.1 to Article 2.10 of the code:

Articles 2.1–2.10 Heterogeneity of ADRVs

2.1 Presence of a Prohibited Substance or its Metabolites or Markers in an Athlete's Sample.

2.2 Use or Attempted Use by an Athlete of a Prohibited Substance or a Prohibited Method.

2.3 Evading Sample Collection.

2.4 Filing Failures and Missed Tests.

2.5 Tampering or Attempted Tampering with any part of Doping Control.

2.6 Possession of a Prohibited Substance or a Prohibited Method.

2.7 Trafficking or Attempted Trafficking in any Prohibited Substance or Prohibited Method.

2.8 Administration or Attempted Administration to any Athlete In-Competition of any Prohibited Method or Prohibited Substance, or Administration or Attempted Administration to any Athlete Out-of-Competition of any Prohibited Method or any Prohibited Substance that is prohibited Out-of-Competition.

2.9 Complicity in an Anti-Doping Rule Violation.

2.10 Prohibited Association.

Only rule 2.1 amounts to the presence of a prohibited substance or its metabolites or markers in the athlete's sample. Contrary to the common-sense view, there is no essence to doping, understood under WADA's official definition of an anti-doping rule violation (ADRV). Rather there are 10 different ways in which an athlete may fall foul of the rules and be banned. Of course, the paradigm case is the ingestion of a substance on the prohibited list, but there are nine other ways of incurring a sanction for an ADRV (many of which do not concern us here; see McNamee 2016; Loland and McNamee 2016). This range of criteria allows anti-doping organisations to capture fully the scope of doping behaviours extending beyond the mere ingestion of banned substances, which is the common-sense understanding of doping. A substance or method will be considered for inclusion in the prohibited list if it meets any two of the following three criteria as outlined in article 4.3.1:

4.3.1.1 Medical or other scientific evidence, pharmacological effect or experience that the substance or method, alone or in combination with other substances or methods, has the potential to enhance or enhances sport performance;

4.3.1.2 Medical or other scientific evidence, pharmacological effect or experience that the Use of the substance or method represents an actual or potential health risk to the Athlete;

4.3.1.3 WADA's determination that the Use of the substance or method violates the spirit of sport described in the introduction to the Code.

The fact that a substance or method meets at least two of the three criteria is a sufficient condition for the substance to be considered for inclusion in the prohibited list. Loland and McNamee (2016) further note that even if the two first criteria are thought of as matters to be settled empirically, applying the criteria in practice is far from straightforward. In 4.3.1.1 and 4.3.1.2 the word 'potential' is used, which opens up factual judgements to considerable interpretation. Not only that, but contrary to the imprecise characterisation offered by Savulescu (2016), WADA does not aim to offer a definition of the spirit of sport. Instead, WADA offers a litany of reasons that it might adduce in arguments about a substance or method being against the spirit of sport, which would (in combination with at least one of the other criteria) be sufficient to place it on the Prohibited List (McNamee 2016).

In addition, there are philosophical questions about what constitutes a 'health risk', and about what kinds and levels of health risks should be deemed to be a concern of anti-doping policy, given that people can take upon themselves many kinds of risks in contexts other than sport. Although WADA acknowledges in its third criterion about the violation of the spirit of sport that the doping debate is ultimately a debate about ethical values, no philosopher is a constituent member of the committee that determines the Prohibited List, which seems an obvious lacuna. This said, although there may be good reasons to challenge the spirit-of-sport criterion, the definition's being 'hopeless' (as Savulescu 2016 asserts) is not one of them. This is simply because WADA does not offer one. What is required is interpretation of the criterion of 'spirit of sport' to determine candidacy for the Prohibited List. But this is required of all the criteria, not just the spirit-of-sport one. Of course, this is fundamentally a philosophical task, which is currently performed by scientists and physicians without training in philosophy, who must determine what constitutes harm or potential harm, performance enhancement or potential performance enhancement. Again, of course, these are fundamentally normative questions that require philosophical consideration. What we must now attempt to do is to consider how criterion 4.3.1.1 regarding (potential) performance enhancement can be interpreted in the light of our extended discussion regarding the distinction between therapy and enhancement.

6.5 Therapy, enhancement and the therapeutic use exemption (TUE) certificate in anti-doping regulations

Examples of challenges to the therapy/enhancement distinction in sports medicine abound. We discuss one recent example as reported by Hamilton and Dimeo.[6] This is the case of cortisol, a steroid that can be prescribed under a therapeutic use exemption (TUE) to facilitate a swifter return to play. Hamilton and Dimeo discuss the case of baseball player Ryan Zimmerman. After injuring his shoulder in the summer of 2012, Zimmerman was able to go from 'being one of baseball's worst hitters to one of its best' thanks, supposedly, to cortisol injections (Hamilton and Dimeo 2015).

Conservative treatment of acute muscle injuries would include rest, ice, elevation, compression, rehabilitation exercises and non-steroidal anti-inflammatory medications (Wong et al. 2015). However, in recent years, advances in understanding of muscle injury physiology and healing have led to proposed adjuvant treatments, such as steroid injections in or around tendons and ligaments. Corticosteroid injections, such as cortisol, can be prescribed under a TUE for swifter return to play after a muscle injury (Rotunno et al. 2016).

We note here, however, that US Anti-Doping Agency (USADA) is not involved in the administration of Major League Baseball (MLB)'s anti-doping programme and they aren't WADA Code signatories. Hence, for Zimmerman, the use of cortisol would have been permissible under the MLB programme with no TUE required.[7] The arguments below, however, are valid nonetheless, as cortisol can be prescribed under a TUE in all other sports regulated by WADA.

WADA have developed an international standard for the issuing of therapies to athletes that might otherwise constitute an ADRV. In constructing such a standard they attempt to steer a middle path between recognising athletes' rights to health-care treatments for legitimate medical conditions, and assuring fair competition. In the 2016 version WADA writes:

> The International Standard for Therapeutic Use Exemptions (ISTUE) was created with the understanding that, due to illness or medical condition, an *Athlete* may require the *Use* of medications or treatments on the World Anti-Doping Agency's *(WADA's) Prohibited List*.
>
> The presence of a *Prohibited Substance* or its *Metabolites* or *Markers*, and/or the *Use* or *Attempted Use, Possession* or *Administration* or *Attempted Administration* of a *Prohibited Substance* or *Prohibited Method* shall not be considered an anti-doping rule violation (ADRV) if it is consistent with the provisions of a Therapeutic Use Exemption (*TUE*) granted in accordance with the ISTUE (*Code* Article 4.4.1).
>
> A *TUE* is granted to an *Athlete* under narrow, well-defined conditions. The *TUE* enables the *Athlete* to take the necessary medication while competing in sport *Events*, without resulting in a doping offence.
>
> The *Athlete* must have a well-documented medical condition, backed up by reliable, relevant and sufficient medical data (ISTUE Article 6.2) that demonstrate he/she meets the criteria for grant of a *TUE*. This mandatory documentation supports the *Athlete's TUE* application to his/her relevant *Anti-Doping Organization (ADO)*.[8]

The principle behind the policy is ethically defensible: an athlete ought not to forgo legitimate treatments for medical conditions just to compete in sport, and the TUE protects their right to healthcare. The application of the principle is, however, open to considerable abuse. Cortisol is a powerful drug. It allows the body to utilise stored energy in the muscles, liver and fat tissue. It does not heal the injury, but allows the athlete to play through it, although not without long-term consequences. We know that steroids can have long-term implications for the health of the athlete, including the risk of tendon or fascial rupture following corticosteroid injections (Wong et al. 2015; Rotunno et al. 2016), and other cardiovascular complications (Angell et al. 2012).

Drugs prescribed for return to play, such as cortisol, are good examples of drugs that confer a performance advantage. This performance advantage can be compared to the advantage conferred by a performance-enhancing drug like testosterone, which is included in the WADA Prohibited List. Testosterone is rarely, if ever, prescribed under a TUE (with the only exceptions being in some sports such as power lifting and bodybuilding, that have non-tested federations), even though its anabolic steroid effects are very similar to the one produced by cortisol, as they have a very similar chemical structure.

It is difficult to estimate the prevalence of doping. According to a recent article by Ulrich et al. (2017), the estimated prevalence of doping at the 13th IAAF Athletics World Championships in Daegu, South Korea in August 2011 and at the 12th Quadrennial Pan-Arab Games (PAG) in Doha, Qatar in December 2011 was respectively 43.6% (95% confidence interval 39.4–47.9) and 57.1% (95% confidence interval 52.4–61.8) (Ulrich et al. 2017). It is widely believed that athletes are willing to sacrifice their long-term health for short-term goals and competitive advantages on the field of play. Most evidence is anecdotal, and certainly the famous Goldman study that is often cited, concerning those who would take a drug that would win an Olympic medal while curtailing their lives, is methodologically problematic (Goldman et al. 1984). Nevertheless, there is more recent evidence that this assumption has merit (Krumer et al. 2011) and the widespread belief supports paternalistic practices in anti-doping. Should athletes under a bio-liberal doping policy be allowed to take drugs such as cortisol, which can have long-lasting effects on their health, in the expectation of a swifter return to play?

An attempt to analyse the problem of the use of corticosteroids for a swifter return to play will require the application of the therapy/enhancement distinction. WADA has four criteria for the protocol of awarding a TUE certificate, and we make suppositions in relation to them. So, let us suppose (having no confidential medical notes to work from) that due process has satisfactorily resolved 'on the balance of probabilities' (which is the quasi-jurisprudential test) that athlete Z has 'a significant impairment to health if the *Prohibited Substance* or *Prohibited Method* were to be withheld'.[9] Let us also assume, second, that 'The Therapeutic *Use* of the *Prohibited Substance* or *Prohibited Method* is highly unlikely to produce any additional enhancement of performance beyond what might be anticipated by a return to the *Athlete's* normal state of health'. Note here that one need not have made any mistakes in reasonably anticipating such enhancement of performance, contrary to the facts upon athlete Z's return to play. Third, 'There is no reasonable Therapeutic alternative' and finally, in keeping with WADA protocol, the need for the TUE does not arise 'wholly or in part, to prior *Use* (without a *TUE*) of a substance or method that was prohibited at the time of such *Use*'. What ought we think of the ethical justifiability of a (series of) cortisol injections?

It is interesting to note how the anabolic steroid testosterone (which, as noted above, has a very similar chemical structure and effects as cortisol, and is considered a performance-enhancing drug for which rarely, if ever, TUE are granted) can and is indeed prescribed outside the sports context as 'therapy for hypogonadism'. Under such circumstances, athlete Z appears to be justified in seeking to being granted the TUE. Interestingly the former Olympic and professional British cyclist Chris Boardman suffers from precisely such a defect, and this is thought to be evidence of his riding the Tour de France and other such debilitating touring races under testosterone-depleting circumstances (Hamilton and Dimeo 2015).

Hypogonadism by definition can include a variety of conditions, since it is defined as 'a condition in which the body doesn't produce enough testosterone – the hormone that plays a key role in masculine growth and development during puberty – or has an impaired ability to produce sperm or both'.[10] Hypogonadism can be an inborn condition or develop later in life and signs and symptoms may vary to include one or more of the following symptoms (with different degrees of severity): erectile dysfunction, infertility, decrease in body hair growth and muscle mass, development of breast tissue (gynecomastia) and loss of bone mass (osteoporosis).

The prescription of testosterone to an individual affected by hypogonadism, in order to restore him to a previous or normal species functioning 'state of health', seems to be part of common medical practice. But the definition of hypogonadism itself is not fixed and can be changed to provide a different benchmark of 'normality' that needs to be restored. Moreover, as we have noted, one and the same pharmacology may be therapeutic for one population, enhancing for another and/or both for the same pathological population. Alexis Madrigal (2015) reports that nearly 4% of men in their 60s in the US are using testosterone. The number of men between 40 and 64 went up 77% from 2010 to 2013 in the USA, to 1.5 million men. Madrigal notes that the emerging popularity of testosterone has opened up whole new business models for entrepreneurial doctors. It seems, therefore, that we are left to conclude that the same drug can be prescribed legally within the context of medicine to restore a former state of health (or because of its enhancing effects?), but not within the context of sport because of its performance-enhancing effects.

Indeed, Hamilton and Dimeo seem to hint at this when they write that the use of testosterone to treat 'real medical problems' and anti-ageing (where the latter are not considered 'real' medical problems) has increased globally, as reported by an Australian study (Handelsman 2013; also reported in Hamilton and Dimeo 2015). The alleged distinction between real and less real medical problems presupposes a reference to a 'health' state defined naturalistically as biostatistically normal functioning. But we have noted how what counts as biostatistically normal functioning is in part contingent on social contexts and includes value judgements about a 'normal' male performance relative to age. While Hamilton and Dimeo seem to imply that Zimmerman's recovery is incredible (literally, unbelievable) we have offered a therapeutic scenario in which a TUE could legitimately be offered. Clearly, there is an issue concerning the foreseeability of enhancing, which the second criterion aims to rule out. Interestingly, Zimmerman himself points to a non-cortisol reductionist story which is at least plausible:

I'm OK with the slow starts, but not being able to swing the bat and do the things health-wise, I was worried about that. Because I know my body pretty well. Everyone in this room plays hurt. Everyone in every locker room. Nobody's healthy. And I've played hurt a lot just like everyone else. But it was a different kind of feeling. It made me nervous.

That was a trying time, I guess you could say. That was about as tough a six-week stretch as I've ever had in my career. To be able to look up there now and know I've been able to battle back from that – and more importantly, can actually help the team win now – I'm pretty proud of it.[11]

Now it is of course possible that we could be naive in our reading. On the one hand, the athlete could be taking other substances that are on the Prohibited List, but it would be difficult to see how such a change in medication might bring about such a tangible improvement by pharmacological means alone. On the other hand we might see that a genuine problem, a medicated response, the placebo effect, less tension-fuelled protection of the joint when swinging, and so on and so forth, might contribute to the dramatic improvement. One journalistic source writes of Zimmerman's story:

> One of the worst hitters in baseball before the cortisone injection and one of the best hitters in baseball since the cortisone injection, which is doubly remarkable considering at the time doctors told Zimmerman that they weren't sure how much good the shot would do on his shoulder.
>
> *(Gleeman 2012)*

This piece of pharmacological reductionism – implying that the drug or hormone alone was sufficient for the performance enhancement – is certainly no more credible than our rendering of the batting progress of Zimmerman. And of course, it might just be that the process itself was corrupted, and there was no such condition in the first place. But that would be one big conspiracy story.

In contrast to what might be seen as a permissive stance towards the therapy/ enhancement distinction, let us discuss another example, this time from the world of Paralympic sport. Consider the Court of Arbitration for Sport (CAS) ruling on the International Paralympic Committee (IPC) versus the 52-year-old paraplegic shooter Warren Berger (2010), who needed beta-blockers for a serious heart condition. He had used the drug Metropolol for many years. The drug is on the Prohibited List and is neither available to athletes in or out of completion. Nevertheless, the IPC refused to issue a TUE certificate on the basis that the medication for which clearance was sought would be performance enhancing to the extent that it would challenge the integrity of the competition.

In the Paralympic sport case many TUEs are sought by virtue of the impaired population. Yet in this case we find a stronger line taken than that by WADA, other things being equal. Here the right to healthcare was not denied. Rather the IPC held that the athlete was ineligible to enter the competition while taking the drug. Though Berger sought redress at the CAS, the ruling against issuing a TUE was denied by IPC and the CAS upheld it. The ruling stated:

> Considering the medical evidence as a whole, we take the view the appellant has not demonstrated that the therapeutic use of the Prohibited Substance would produce no additional enhancement of performance other than that which might be anticipated by return to a state of normal health following the treatment of a legitimate medical condition. Thus we have reached the conclusion that the athlete in this case, at this time, on the basis of all the evidence before us, has not discharged the burden resting upon him to establish his entitlement to a TUE for the use of Metoprolol whilst participating in his chosen sport of shooting.[12]

There are doubtless thousands of cases where TUEs are granted or not granted. And not only may different authorities – national federations, international federations, IPC, WADA etc. – grant them on different bases, but they may very well agree on the facts or disagree on them. They may well accept that a medical condition is present and fail to approve a drug on the Prohibited List or they may well agree that it meets the conditions to be granted one, where it is not wholly certain what if any the performance-enhancing effect might be.[13]

6.6 Conclusions

This chapter is in a sense the hinge of the book. We have discussed a series of genetically related issues concerning medicine, medical research and medical technology. Many of these discussions have charted contentious bioethical positions that we have mapped on to realistic sports scenarios. This chapter has had to deal head-on with two problems. The first, the therapy/enhancement distinction, is an issue that has brought great division at the biopolitical fault lines of bioethics. It has also taken an enormously problematic aspect of anti-doping policy, the granting of TUE certifications for medications on the prohibited list, and shown how no theory-neutral answer to the justifiability of their issuance is available.

Our discussion of the goals of medicine and sports medicine first alerted us to that difficulty. Sports medicine professionals and official definitions are traditionally aligned to therapeutic and preventative aims. Yet sports medicine practice in elite sport, at least, aims at optimising performance. WADA policy appears to demand a restrictive account of sports medicine. By contrast bioliberal writers in medicine and sports medicine adopt a model of medicine that is person-centred (some would say, customer-focused), and acknowledges the enhancement aim as a legitimate aspect of medicine, not least because in many cases it cannot be separated from therapeutic practice. Each clearly brings different values into play, and some coherent rationale is required to explain the differences, if they are thought to be legitimate.

When disputing matters of enhancement, criteria beyond mere individual choice must be borne in mind (Holm and McNamee 2009; Camporesi 2014). For present purposes, we might benefit from considering the broader goals of sport and society (Parens 1998;

Douglas 2007), the narrower goals of biomedicine (Juengst 1998), and the ethics of self-improvement (ibid.), including the dignity of human activity (Kass 2003). Juengst, by way of warning, writes that 'For policy makers faced with the prospect of using enhancement as a regulatory concept it will be important to have a clear map of these uses and interpretations' (Juengst 1998, 29). If it is true that the therapy/enhancement distinction can only be evaluated on its application in a case by case basis, then we should know more about the state of the science underpinning each, and consider these in relation to the contexts of sports. We shall proceed to do this in the following chapters.

Notes

All websites accessed October 2017.

1 A portion of Section 6.2 was previously published in Camporesi, S. (2014). *From Bench to Bedside, to Track & Field: The Context of Enhancement and its Ethical Relevance*. San Francisco, CA: University of California Medical Humanities Press. ISBN: 978-0-9889865-4-1. We would like to acknowledge Professor Brian Dolan, Editor of UC Medical Humanities Press, for granting us permission to use the content in this volume. We also would like to acknowledge Jim Parry for giving us helpful feedback on this chapter.

2 www.bbc.com/sport/athletics/22269445

3 Though it recently morphed into the field of sport and exercise medicine. The British-based Faculty for Sport and Exercise Medicine writes: 'Sport and Exercise Medicine involves the medical care of injury and illness in sport and exercise and has a large scale application in improving the health of the general public through exercise advice and prescription.' (www.fsem.ac.uk/about-us.aspx)

4 To be fair that line of argument is first laid out by Thomas Murray as early as 1983, and has been refashioned by many authors in the philosophy of sport since (Murray, T. H. (1983). The coercive power of drugs in sports. Hastings Center Report, 13(4), 24–30).

5 www.wada-ama.org/en/resources/the-code/world-anti-doping-code

6 Another example which came to our attention during the proof stages of the book is reported by Andrew Till: www.outsideonline.com/2187821/accidental-doper

7 Many thanks to Matt Fedoruk for alerting us to this point (personal communication, 26 July, 2017).

8 www.wada-ama.org/sites/default/files/resources/files/wada-tue-guidelines-v8.0-en.pdf

9 See www.wada-ama.org/sites/default/files/resources/files/wada-2015-world-anti-doping-code.pdf

10 Mayo definition of hypogonadism: www.mayoclinic.org/diseases-conditions/male-hypogonadism/symptoms-causes/dxc-20248457

11 http://mlb.nbcsports.com/2012/09/13/cortisone-injection-saved-ryan-zimmermans-season/

12 http://arbitrationlaw.com/files/free_pdfs/CAS%202009-A-1948%20RB%20v%20WADA%20Award.pdf

13 Of course there is always the placebo effect, where athletes can be granted a TUE that e.g. WADA consider non-enhancing, but which has that effect for them because of their subjective beliefs.

References

All websites accessed October 2017.

Abrahams, Adolphe. 1958. The use and abuse of drugs by athletes. *Addiction*, 55(1): 23–28. doi:10.1111/j.1360-0443.1958.tb05458.x

Allert, G., B. Blasszauer, K. Boyd and D. Callahan. 1996. The goals of medicine: setting new priorities. *The Hastings Center Report*, 26(6): S1.

Angell, P.J., N. Chester, N. Sculthorpe, G. Whyte, K. George and J. Somauroo. 2012. Performance enhancing drug abuse and cardiovascular risk in athletes: implications for the clinician. *British Journal of Sports Medicine*, 46 (Suppl 1): i78–i84.

Barnes, J., J.A.K. Thompson and H. Tredennick. 1976. *The Ethics of Aristotle: The Nicomachean Ethics*. England: Penguin Books.

Berryman, J.W. and R.J. Park, eds. 1992. *Sport and Exercise Science: Essays in the History of Sports Medicine*. Urbana, IL: University of Illinois Press.

Boorse, C. 1977. Health as a theoretical concept. *Philosophy of Science*, 44(4): 542–573.

Boorse, C. 1997. A rebuttal on health. In *What is disease?*, eds J.M. Humber and R.F. Almeder. Totowa, NJ: Humana Press, pp. 1–134.

Buchanan, A., D.W. Brock, N. Daniels and D. Wikler. 2001. *From Chance to Choice: Genetics and Justice*. Cambridge: Cambridge University Press.

Camporesi, S. 2014. *From Bench to Bedside, to Track & Field: The Context of Enhancement and its Ethical Relevance*. London: UC Medical Humanities Press.

Camporesi, S. and M.J. McNamee. 2014. Performance enhancement, elite athletes and anti doping governance: comparing human guinea pigs in pharmaceutical research and professional sports. *Philosophy, Ethics, and Humanities in Medicine*, 9(1): 4.

Carter, N. 2013. The origins of British sports medicine, 1850–1914. *Gesnerus*, 70(1): 17–35.

Daniels, N. 2000. Normal functioning and the treatment-enhancement distinction. *Cambridge Quarterly of Healthcare Ethics*, 9(3): 309–322.

Der Spiegel. 1987. Rutschbahn in den legalen Drogensumpf. Available at: www.spiegel.de/spiegel/print/d-13523874.html

Dimeo, P. 2007. A critical assessment of John Hoberman's histories of drugs in sport. *Sport in History*, 27(2): 318–342.

Douglas, T. 2007. Enhancement in sport, and enhancement outside sport. *Studies in Ethics, Law, and Technology*, 1(1): Article 2. doi:10.2202/1941-6008.1000

Edwards, S.D. and M. McNamee. 2006. Why sports medicine is not medicine. *Health Care Analysis*, 14(2): 103–109.

Eilers, M., K. Grüber and C. Rehmann-Sutter, eds. 2014. *The Human Enhancement Debate and Disability: New Bodies for a Better Life*. Houndmills: Palgrave MacMillan.

Engelhardt Jr, H.T. (1990). The birth of the medical humanities and the rebirth of the philosophy of medicine: the vision of Edmund D. Pellegrino. *The Journal of Medicine and Philosophy*, 15(3): 237–241.

Foddy, B. and J. Savulescu. 2007. Ethics of performance enhancement in sport: drugs and gene doping. In *Principles of Health Care Ethics*, eds R.E. Ashcroft, A. Dawson, H. Draper and J. McMillan, 2nd edn, pp. 511–519. Chichester, England: John Wiley and Sons, pp. 511–519.

Gleaves, J. and M. Llewellyn. 2014. Sport, drugs and amateurism: tracing the real cultural origins of anti-doping rules in international sport. *The International Journal of the History of Sport*, 31(8): 839–853.

Gleeman, A. 2012. Cortisone injection saved Ryan Zimmerman's season. *NBC Sports*. Available at: http://mlb.nbcsports.com/2012/09/13/cortisone-injection-saved-ryan-zimmermans-season/

Goldman, B., P.J. Bush and R. Klatz. 1984. *Death in the Locker Room*. South Bend, IN: Icarus Press.

Green, S.K. 2004. Discussion: practice makes perfect? Ideal standards and practice norms in sports. *Virtual Mentor*, 6(7). Available at http://journalofethics.ama-assn.org/2004/07/jdsc1-0407.html

Hamilton, L. and P. Dimeo. 2015. Steroids in sport: zero tolerance to testosterone needs to change. *The Conversation*. Available at https://theconversation.com/steroids-in-sport-zer o-tolerance-to-testosterone-needs-to-change-48774

Handelsman, D.J. 2013. Global trends in testosterone prescribing, 2000–2011: expanding the spectrum of prescription drug misuse. *Medical Journal of Australia*, 199(8): 548–551.

Harris, J. 2010. *Enhancing Evolution: The Ethical Case for Making Better People*. Princeton, NJ: Princeton University Press.

Harvey, R. 1988. Steroids were not an answer for Heptathlete: West Germany's Dressel died at 26 from using performance-enhancing drug. *Los Angeles Times*, 18 July. Available at: http://articles.latimes.com/1988-07-18/sports/sp-4362_1_west-germany

Heggie, V. 2011. *A History of British Sports Medicine*. Manchester: Manchester University Press.

Hoberman, J. 1992. *Mortal Engines. The Science of Performance and the Dehumanization of Sport*. New York: The Free Press.

Hoberman, J. 2014. Physicians and the sports doping epidemic. *Virtual Mentor*, 16(7): 570–574.

Holm, S. and M. McNamee. 2009. Ethics in sports medicine. *British Medical Journal*, 339: b3898.

Holm, S. and M. McNamee. 2011. Physical enhancement: what baseline, whose judgment? In *Enhancing Human Capacities*, eds J. Savulescu, R. ter Meulen and G. Kahane. Hoboken, NJ: John Wiley & Sons, pp. 291–303.

Johnson, R. 2004. The unique ethics of sports medicine. *Clinics in Sports Medicine*, 23(2): 175–182.

Jonas, H. 1974. *Philosophical Essays: From Ancient Creed to Technological Man*. Englewood Cliffs, NJ: Prentice Hall.

Juengst, E.T. 1998. What does enhancement mean. In *Enhancing Human Traits: Ethical and Social Implications*, ed. E. Parens. Washington, DC: Georgetown University Press, pp. 29–47.

Kass, L.R. 2003. *Beyond Therapy: Biotechnology and the Pursuit of Happiness*. New York: Dana Press.

Kingma, E. 2007. What is it to be healthy? *Analysis*, 67(2): 128–133.

Kluka, R. 2015. Medicalization, 'normal function' and the definition of health. In *The Routledge Companion to Bioethics*, eds J.D. Arras, E. Fenton and R. Kukla. London: Routledge, pp. 515–530.

Krumer, A., T. Shavit and M. Rosenboim. 2011. Why do professional athletes have different time preferences than non-athletes? *Judgment and Decision Making*, 6(6): 542–551.

Larriviere, D., M.A. Williams, M. Rizzo and R.J. Bonnie. 2009. Responding to requests from adult patients for neuroenhancements: guidance of the Ethics, Law and Humanities Committee. *Neurology*, 73(17): 1406–1412.

Leadbetter, J.D. and W.B. Leadbetter. 1996. The philosophy of sports medicine care: an historical review. *Maryland Medical Journal*, 45(8): 618–631.

Lewens, T. 2015. *The Biological Foundations of Bioethics*. Oxford: OUP.

Loland, S. and M. McNamee. 2016. Anti-doping, performance enhancement, and 'the spirit of sport': a philosophical and ethical critique. In *Doping and Public Health*, eds N. Ahmadi, A. Ljungqvist and G. Svedsäter. Abingdon: Routledge, pp. 111–123.

McNamee, M.J. 2007. Whose Prometheus? Transhumanism, biotechnology and the moral topography of sports medicine. *Sports, Ethics and Philosophy*, 1(2): 181–194.

McNamee, M.J. 2012. The spirit of sport and the medicalisation of anti-doping: empirical and normative ethics. *Asian Bioethics Review*, 4(4): 374–392.

McNamee, M. 2016. Doping scandals, Rio, and the future of anti-doping ethics. Or: what's wrong with Savulescu's recommendations for the regulation of pharmacological enhancement in sport. *Sport, Ethics and Philosophy*, 10(2): 113–116.

McNamee, M.J. and L. Tarasti. 2010. Juridical and ethical peculiarities in doping policy. *Journal of Medical Ethics*, 36(3): 165–169.

Madrigal, A. 2015. Why testosterone is the drug of the future. *Splinter*. Available at: http://splinternews.com/why-testosterone-is-the-drug-of-the-future-1793844976

Mills, C. 2011. *Futures of Reproduction: Bioethics and Biopolitics* (vol. 49). Dordrecht; Heidelberg; London; New York: Springer Science & Business Media.

Mills, C. 2015. Liberal eugenics, human enhancement and the concept of the normal. In *Medicine and Society, New Perspectives in Continental Philosophy*, pp. 179–194. Netherlands: Springer.

Møller, V. 2005. Knud Enemark Jensen's death during the 1960 Rome Olympics: a search for truth? *Sport in History*, 25(3): 452–471.

Murray, T.H. 1983. The coercive power of drugs in sports. *Hastings Center Report*, 13(4): 24–30.

Murray, T.H. 2009. Ethics and endurance-enhancing technologies in sport. In *Performance-Enhancing Technologies in Sports: Ethical, Conceptual, and Scientific Issues*, eds T.H. Murray, K.J. Maschke and A.A. Wasunna. Baltimore: Johns Hopkins University Press, pp. 144–159.

Parens, E. 1998. Is better always good? The enhancement project. *Hastings Center Report*, 28(1): S1–S17.

Ritchie, I. 2014. Pierre de Coubertin, doped 'amateurs' and the 'spirit of sport': the role of mythology in Olympic anti-doping policies. *The International Journal of the History of Sport*, 31(8): 820–838.

Rothman, S.M. and D.J. Rothman. 2003. *The Pursuit of Perfection*. New York: Pantheon.

Rotunno, A., D.J. van Rensburg, C.C. Grant and A.J. van Rensburg. 2016. Corticosteroids in sports-related injuries: friend or foe. *South African Family Practice*, 58(6): 28–33.

Sandel, M. 2004. The case against perfection. *The Atlantic Monthly*, 293(3): 51–62.

Savulescu, J. 2016. Doping scandals, Rio and the future of human enhancement. *Bioethics*, 30(5): 300–303.

Schües, C. 2014. Improving deficiencies? Historical, anthropological, and ethical aspects of the human condition. In *The Human Enhancement Debate and Disability*, eds M. Eilers, K. Grüber and C. Rehmann-Sutter. Houndmills: Palgrave Macmillan, pp. 38–63.

Scully, J.L. 2014. On unfamiliar moral territory: about variant embodiment, enhancement and normativity. In *The Human Enhancement Debate and Disability*, eds M. Eilers, K. Grüber and C. Rehmann-Sutter. Houndmills: Palgrave Macmillan UK, pp. 23–37.

Scully, J.L. and C. Rehmann-Sutter. 2001. When norms normalize: the case of genetic 'enhancement'. *Human Gene Therapy*, 12(1): 87–95.

Time Magazine. 1988. Heptathlete Birgit Dressel: an athlete dying young. Available at: http://content.time.com/time/magazine/article/0,9171,968618,00.html

Ulrich, R., H.G. Pope, L. Cléret et al. 2017. Doping in two elite athletics competitions assessed by randomized-response surveys. *Sports Medicine*. doi:10.1007/s40279-017-0765-4

Williams, J.P.G., ed. 1962. *Sports Medicine*. London: Arnold.

Wong, S., A. Ning, C. Lee and B.T. Feeley. 2015. Return to sport after muscle injury. *Current Reviews in Musculoskeletal Medicine*, 8(2): 168–175.

7

A CASE STUDY IN 'GENE ENHANCEMENT': GENE TRANSFER TO RAISE THE TOLERANCE TO PAIN – A LEGITIMATE MODE OF ENHANCEMENT, OR ILLEGITIMATE DOPING?

7.1 Introduction[1]

In this chapter we explore the question of whether it is ethically justifiable for individuals to seek an experimental gene transfer treatment in order to raise their tolerance to pain. We consider here two plausible scenarios in which an individual is seeking treatment with gene transfer tools to better cope with pain: in the first scenario the individual is a patient; in the second an athlete. We employ a comparative strategy to highlight the similarities and dissimilarities between the ethical frameworks used to evaluate the two scenarios, and to reach conclusions regarding the justifiability of the practice in the two contexts.

Untreatable pain represents an enormous problem to society. As estimated by current statistics, approximately 20 per cent of the adult population suffers from chronic pain, and the financial cost to society is estimated at more than €200 billion per annum in Europe, and $150 billion per annum in the USA (Tracey and Bushnell 2009). Treatment options are limited, with many patients either not responding or having incomplete pain reduction (Breivik et al. 2006). In the last decade, several clinical trials have been carried out using gene transfer tools that aim to overcome this medical need. Gene transfer trials qualify as translational trials, as they are designed to bring to the bedside tools developed at the bench of the molecular biology laboratory. A search performed with keywords 'gene transfer' and 'pain' on the National Health Institutes clinical trials directory revealed ten clinical trials, of which seven are completed, one is active, and two that are either completed or in recruitment.[2] Some of these trials are aimed at treating intractable cancer pain, some at treating pain associated with angina pectoris, others at epidermolysis bullosa (a heritable condition where connective tissue disease causes painful blisters in the skin and mucosal membranes) and others to treat the pain associated with peripheral arterial occlusion (a mini-stroke in the leg which causes the necrosis of muscular tissue, leading to impaired functionality and chronic pain). This last kind of pain, and the related clinical trial (named 'VEGF Gene Transfer for Critical Limb Ischemia', clinical trial identifier NCT00304837), serves as a case study for our comparative evaluation between a medical context and a sports context, where the former is a traditionally conceived therapeutic intervention, and the latter is one where the intervention rests in the grey zone between therapy and enhancement – or as it has been labelled, therapeutic enhancement (Tännsjö 2010).

7.2 Setting the scene: the patient vs the athlete

In scenario (a), the protagonist of the US TV series *House, MD*, Dr Gregory House (played by the British actor Hugh Laurie), has suffered from peripheral ischaemia to his left leg, which has left him limping and with intractable chronic pain, due to the extensive necrotic muscular tissue in his thigh muscles. After having unsuccessfully tried standard and less standard treatments, our protagonist seeks out experimental treatments, i.e. treatments that are currently being tested in clinical trials and not yet approved by national regulatory bodies such as the US Food & Drug Administration (FDA) or the European Medicines Agency (EMA). Among the gene transfer trials currently active or recruiting, one study stands out as the perfect match for a patient like Dr Gregory House. The trial (Identifier # NCT00304837) is a phase 1 study that seeks to transfer the DNA codifying for vascular endothelial growth factor (VEGF) in the legs of patients with peripheral artery disease (PAD). PAD encompasses a range of conditions presenting with blockages in the arteries in the limbs. The nature of the disease is progressive, so that it frequently leads to patients presenting with claudication or critical limb ischemia (CLI), exactly the manifestations which are present in Dr Gregory House (Mughal et al. 2012).

Most phase 1 studies are designed to test the safety of a new pharmaceutical or other treatment in a restricted number of patients, after the treatment has proved efficacious in laboratory testing and animal models, but some – like this one – may also test the efficacy of the substance under study. This particular trial aims not only at testing the safety of VEGF-gene transfer, but also at improving rest pain and/or healing the ulcers caused by PAD. According to the trial protocol, the DNA codifying for the vascular endothelial growth factor (VEGF) protein is injected into the affected legs of the trial subjects on three separate occasions, each two weeks apart. The DNA codifier then directs the cells of the artery wall to increase production of VEGF, which has been shown to cause new blood vessels to grow around the blockages in the leg arteries (Mughal et al. 2012). It has also been demonstrated that increased VEGF expression through gene transfer techniques improves microcirculation in muscle, and hence increased oxygen and nutrient supply, as well as removal of waste products (Giacca and Zacchigna 2012). Kim et al. have observed evidence of growth of new collateral vessels, relief of ischaemic pain and ulcer healing in patients with CLI (Kim et al. 2004)

Generally speaking, as we noted in Chapter 5 in this volume, there are two kinds of safety concerns about gene transfer. These relate both to the kind of carrier/vector being used (usually a modified virus) and to the encoded transgene. In our case study, the former (vector) risks are eliminated by injecting the DNA coding for the VEGF protein directly into the patients' leg muscles, without any viral or non-viral carrier. This eliminates the risks inherent in the vectors and common to many other gene transfer trials. As to the latter risks, it has been shown that overexpression of VEGF causes haemangiomas (benign tumours characterised by an increased number of vessels) in skeletal muscle in mouse animal models (Springer et al. 1998). In addition, angiogenesis can have detrimental consequences in non-target tissues. Transient peripheral oedema (swelling) due to increased local perfusion is a relatively common and mild side effect. In addition, the theoretical risk of facilitation of tumour vascularisation (and therefore, increased growth) or plaque angiogenesis in non-target tissues must not be ignored (Baumgartner 2000). More serious adverse effects have been rarely observed and are mostly related to the use of viral vectors, and therefore are not pertinent to the trial we are discussing, which injects DNA in the form of a plasmid (a circular molecule of DNA) (Muona et al. 2012). A recent study conducted by Muona and co-authors and aimed at assessing the long-term side effects (10+ years) of local VEGF gene transfer to ischaemic lower limbs found that adenovirus or plasmid (our case) or liposome mediated intravascular local gene transfer does not increase the risk of malignancies, diabetes or any other disease in the long term. They also identified, as a key element to safe gene transfer, the local delivery to the treatment site (as in our case study), which reduced the risk of systematic spread of the vector, as well of adverse side effects to other organs. This suggests that the technique described here could be safely applied both in trial subjects and in healthy individuals (which is pertinent to scenario (b), below).

As noted by Mughal et al. (2012), PAD cannot be attributed to one specific genetic cause, and greater therapeutic efficacy could be obtained by targeted gene transfer using multiple growth factors. Indeed, angiogenic gene transfer strategies such as VEGF gene transfer are by no means the only ones being explored in the treatment of chronic pain (Goins et al. 2012), but appear to be among the most advanced at the clinical level, while other strategies are still at the level of animal studies. As a general remark, while we are aware that a certain degree of speculation is necessary when applying our case study to the second scenario (the elite sports context), we think there is sufficient scientific and medical evidence to argue that gene transfer for pain has very plausible applications for enhancing athletic performances.

Our second scenario is less complex, as it does not involve any complex pathology. Thus in scenario (b), our would-be protagonist is an elite athlete competing in an endurance event, such as cross-country skiing, marathon running, tour cycling, triathlon or an event of similar extended duration, seeking VEGF-gene transfer in order to cope better with the pain inherent in the activity. The growth of blood vessels in the limbs, as demonstrated by the clinical trial described above, is likely to aid athletes in their performance by increasing the oxygen carrying capacity to the limbs (nutrient supply) and the removal of waste products. It is also obvious that an athlete feeling less pain could perform better, *ceteris paribus*, than other athletes suffering for their sporting goals.

7.3 Comparing the scenarios

How are we to understand the similarities and differences these contexts present? And to what extent is the ethical permissibility of the practice dependent upon or independent of the context of gene transfer? We respond to these questions by spelling out two ethical frameworks that might be adopted in order to analyse the two scenarios.

Scenario (a): ethics of translational research

Generally, we do not regard pain as a valuable part of our lives. On the contrary, we take measures to diminish or even eliminate pain from our daily lives, and from the lives of those who are dear to us. Even in illnesses where pain is present, we try to eliminate it, although it may not be possible to cure the patient of the underlying cause. Palliative care, which we consider an essential part of treating a sick human being with dignity, is predicated on such an understanding.

The first framework we use to analyse the scenarios is (a) the 'ethics of translational research' approach developed by Jonathan Kimmelman (Kimmelman 2010). Kimmelman develops the new concept of 'translational distance', which refers to the space created between cutting-edge biomedical research and clinical applications. This novel concept, he argues, is necessary as it may not be possible in first-in-human studies to apply the concept of 'clinical equipoise', as defined by Freedman as 'a state of honest, professional disagreement in the community of experts about the preferred treatment' (Freedman 1987). This is because the level of uncertainty is so high in 'first-in' human research employing gene transfer techniques that the robust epistemic and ethical threshold required for clinical equipoise cannot be secured. In its place, the concept of translational distance is a useful kind of 'epistemic heuristic' to understand the bidirectional flow of knowledge between the bench and the bedside, and back. While traditionally the value of early clinical trials has been regarded only in terms of their 'progressive value' towards later phase 2 and phase 3 studies, such a framework is not applicable when evaluating the social value of first-in-human research as in our case study. In Kimmelman's model, phase 1 translational studies between the 'bench and the bedside' are loaded with epistemic value if they stimulate preclinical research or if they stimulate further clinical development. In addition, adopting a translational distance model with a non-progressive epistemic value for these trials would help to dispel the 'therapeutic misconception' (Henderson et al. 2006; Horng and Grady 2003) widespread among (often desperate) first-in clinical trials volunteers.

Therapeutic misconception arises where subjects misinterpret the primary purpose of a clinical trial as therapeutic, and conflate the goals of research with the goals of clinical care. As shown in a study of consent documents of gene transfer clinical trials, 20 per cent of consent documents for gene transfer trials fail to explain their purpose as establishing safety and dosage, while only 41 per cent of oncology trials identify palliative care as an alternative to participation. Moreover, the term 'gene therapy' is used with twice the frequency of the term 'gene transfer' (Kimmelman and Levenstadt 2005). As defined by Kimmelman, the concept of translational distance 'is intended to prompt researchers, review committees, and policy-makers to contemplate the size of the "inferential gap" separating completed preclinical studies and projected human trial results' (Kimmelman 2010, 118) and should inform both the design of the studies (which need to incorporate endpoints that make it possible for the knowledge produced to have an impact in terms of further research) and the ethical approval of the trial.

We agree that Kimmelman's model better captures the reality of how information flows in translational research. As for the individual seeking to be enrolled in such an experimental trial, notwithstanding the model of consent adopted (as set out in Chapter 4), we recommend that researchers spell out the potential risks and benefits of the experimental procedure to the would-be volunteer. Researchers should also evaluate the severity of the pre-existing condition in the subject and its refractoriness to other standard treatments; and they should evaluate the subject's decisional autonomy, which will be predicated on reasonable comprehension (and voluntariness) in relation to the foregoing.

Returning to our fictional protagonist, Dr Gregory House, we can see that in this particular case the risks inherent in gene transfer trials due to the viral vectors are eliminated by injecting VEGF directly into the leg muscles of the patients, and therefore the translational distance between the bench and the bedside can also be considered a modest 'inferential gap'. In addition, the pre-existing condition of chronic pain caused by peripheral artery ischaemia is severe and refractory to standard treatment. Finally, Dr Gregory House seems to be in a position to make an autonomous decision, unclouded by therapeutic misconception. Indeed, Dr House can perhaps be seen as a contemporary instance of the archetypical mythological figure of the 'wounded healer' Chiron, who is able to heal others but unable to heal himself. As autonomy plays a fundamental role in the ethical framework describing the medical context, there would need to be strong reasons to justify interference with the patient's self-regarding and autonomous choice to participate in the trial, even recognising – as we do – that the patient may have no available option (apart from palliative care) other than participating in the trial, due to the severity of his condition and the unavailability of therapeutic options. Provided that all the above conditions were met, we might reasonably reach the conclusion that his informed consent to participating in the VEGF-clinical trial would be valid.

Scenario (b): ethics of sports enhancement

How should we frame the request of an athlete seeking VEGF-gene transfer for the purposes of better coping with pain during a competition? In the first instance, his participation might look like a case of what we could call 'physician-assisted doping'. As discussed in the previous chapter, the World Anti-Doping Agency (WADA) sets out three criteria to classify a product or process as 'doping' (WADA 2015). These pertain to (i) the (potential) performance-enhancing effects; (ii) the potential harm to health; (iii) the (potential) threat to the spirit of sport. Only two criteria need apply for a product or process to be prohibited. The anti-doping code recognises the rights of athletes to secure healthcare, and this right may supersede anti-doping regulations when (as we saw in the previous chapter) specific conditions apply. This does not, however, allow the patient-athlete *carte blanche*. Prior to utilising banned products or processes athletes on a registered testing pool (who are on notice that they may be randomly tested) must submit a Therapeutic Use Exemption (TUE) certificate signed by a relevant medical authority. Retrospective applications are typically frowned upon, but under particular conditions they may be acceptable.

The TUE certifies that the therapy is necessary for the athlete's condition and that no other alternative is available. Though the procedure is in principle robust, clearly, it is open to abuse from 'friendly' doctors prepared to assign a pathological condition that does not exist, or by positing a syndrome for which there is no clear aetiology. Leaving aside for the present the added complexities of unethical behaviour, let us assume that our athlete is asking for a TUE from the relevant authority. In addition to the WADA, this might be an international federation, such as the International Association of Athletics Federations (IAAF), or an event organiser such as the International Olympic Committee (IOC) or the International Paralympic Committee (IPC), who have hitherto taken exclusive charge of in-competition testing during the Olympic and Paralympic Games. There is very little to suggest that a TUE would be achievable in this scenario. Despite TUE precedents for beta-blockers in relation to cardiac patient-athletes in target-accuracy events (such as archery), it is highly unlikely that a TUE would be given for mere pain relief where that pain is simply a marker for injury (and where there may be performance enhancement side effects).[3] Dr Hans Geyer, the deputy director of the World Anti Doping Laboratory in Cologne, widely recognised as one of the premier testing laboratories, remarked upon the practice of using analgesics as analogous to doping: 'It is a grey zone. In my opinion pain killers fulfil all requirements of a doping substance because normally pain is a protection mechanism of the body and with pain killers you switch off this protection system' (McGrath 2012).

Given the long-standing routine use and abuse of painkillers in elite sport (Broglio et al. 2017; Huizenga 1995; Nixon 1992; Nixon 1993), it might be argued that the introduction of VEGF would represent merely an extension of everyday practice. In both the first and the second scenarios, consideration would have to be given to the autonomy of the decision-making of the individual in reaching an ethically justifiable intervention. In the second scenario, this would be thought necessary, while in the first scenario this might be thought both necessary and sufficient, provided that the conditions for a modest translational distance were met, as they are in our case study. Why then is it insufficient in the context of elite sports? Well, in addition to determining the conditions of consent, additional factors regarding the ethical permissibility of VEGF-gene transfer in an athletic context must be considered.

In contrast to scenario (a), pain can be seen as an essential, integral and valuable part of endurance sports. Performing at an elite level in endurance sport and not experiencing pain are mutually exclusive. Indeed, an athlete's ability to tolerate pain is one of the fundamental characteristics that determine athletic performance and provide competitive advantage. Lance Armstrong famously called the Tour de France 'an exercise in pointless suffering' (Fry 2006). He and others have talked insightfully about wanting to take opponents (metaphorically) to existential places that they could not endure (Hamilton and Coyle 2013). The capacity to endure high levels of pain over significant time (i.e. suffering) is a highly prized trait in multi-day/week tour event cycling. Indeed one may refer to them as 'communities of suffering' (McNamee 2008). Not only is it the case that we must distinguish the experience of pain from suffering (Cassell 1998), in sports (Lurie 2006; McNamee 2006), but in addition there are, of course, different kinds of pain an athlete can experience in competition (Koessler 2006). One is the acute, intense and specific pain that occurs suddenly, frequently a result of injury, and is often experienced by athletes competing in football or other contact sports. One can experience such pain in endurance events too – the cycle crash, the herniated disc in running and so on. VEGF-gene transfer treatment would be meaningless for this kind of pain, so it is irrelevant to this discussion. Rather, we wish to discuss the kind of pain that occurs during endurance exercise. This may include muscle soreness or a burning sensation in the lungs, the feeling that one's heart will explode if the same level of intense effort is maintained much longer, and so forth. The strength of these sensations can range from unpleasant to what is typically thought of as unbearable pain. This second kind of pain is typical of endurance sports such as marathons, triathlon, long-distance swimming and cycling, cross-country skiing and so on. Among athletes, the former kind of pain is often referred to as a 'bad' kind, as it impairs the ability of the athlete to continue playing or competing, while the latter is referred to as a 'good' kind of pain, as it pushes the athlete to compete and perform at a higher level. Indeed, many athletes regard this second or 'good kind' of pain as an achievement, and as an essential part of their life and identity as elite athletes (Howe 2004).

The level of physical training of athletes can raise the level of pain that they are able to endure, and make a difference in their performance. Athletes also report that the level of their 'mental toughness' (Crust 2007; Gucciardi et al. 2009) makes a difference in their ability to cope with pain. Different individuals, though, start from very different baselines in their abilities to endure pain (Dolgin 2010), and this is one of the factors, among many other biological and environmental factors, that affect an athlete's performance. Among the other factors that do so are their birthplace (contrast pre-athletic life at altitude, and how this affects phenotypic factors, with competitors born at or near sea level); wealth and other non-athletic factors that can enhance the possibilities of success (contrast athletes or teams with and without sports psychological services, or sponsorships that improve equipment access); and genetic conditions that may confer an advantage over fellow athletes. We have discussed some of these contingent non-biological factors such as birthplace in Chapter 3 (in relation to our discussion of 'talent'), and will discuss genetic and biological advantages in Chapters 8 and 9 in this volume.

7.4 Discussion: levelling out relevant inequalities?

There is no official policy nor widely shared standard for sports administrators or regulatory bodies like WADA to shape discussions on how one might go about levelling out genetic and biological differences to reach a sufficiently 'level playing field' for all athletes: some inequalities are systematically excluded, while others are ignored (Loland and McNamee 2000; Loland 2003). What happens in practice is that we do not usually try to level out biological and genetic factors affecting athletic performance, even where we know that those factors confer an advantage (think of Finnish skier Mäntyranta, discussed in Chapter 5), although there has been a lively discussion about the IAAF policies which exclude women athletes with hyperandrogenism from competing in women's events on the basis of a supposed unfair advantage derived from increased levels of testosterone (see Chapter 8 for a thorough discussion of this case). Typically, philosophers of sport generally agree that the question centres around notions of fairness and equal opportunity, or what Loland calls Fair Opportunity (Loland 2009; Loland and Hoppeler 2012).[4]

Let us think counterfactually here: if we were to try to equalise all the starting conditions (of which tolerance to pain is, again, merely one example) we would move in the direction of having all athletes crossing the finish line at the same point, and then what would be left of the meaning of sport and athletic performance? After all we are precisely interested in distinguishing among relatively excellent (i.e. relevant to a particular class or group), and absolutely excellent performers and performances.

Some sports owe their very existence to gambling, such as jai alai and horse racing (Forrest and Simmons 2003), while others were driven to codify their rules on the basis of the need for bookmakers to have a fair and reliable contest, such as cricket and golf in 1744 (Munting 1996). The practice of handicapping, by adding weights to the favoured horses, appears to owe its existence to the need for tight contests where there was a reasonable chance for any horse to win the race and thereby maximise bookmakers' opportunity to make a profit. The rationale for handicapping also has a place in pedagogical sport, where competitors with significantly varying athletic capabilities may still enjoy a close contest. In other competition structured scenarios, where a league system – again heavily underwritten by commercial media interests – has a strong incentive to prolong interests and more broadly spread opportunities to win, we find systems where lower teams gain access to the best new potential players in a draft system (such as in American football). In skiing, advantages of superior downhill skiers may be manipulated in some competitions by having them go at the end of the run when the snow is at its slowest (Hämäläinen 2013). And in European football (soccer) we see the development of financial fair play regulations to avoid clubs going into deep operating losses (underwritten by high net worth individuals), but also to keep alive uncertainty of outcome by preventing extremely wealthy clubs from buying an amount of athletic talent likely to usurp the competitive possibilities of the league by removing an excessive amount of uncertainty of outcome (Schubert and Könecke 2015).

In each of these cases we see structures of competition or economic considerations arranged so that ethically valuable goals – fair opportunity to contest the goal and uncertainty of outcome – are preserved. The dominant position, therefore, does not include levelling out the effects of the genetic lottery in sports. Other things being equal, more prosaic solutions arise. Thus, if an athlete is likely to achieve a maximum height of 1 metre 40 we steer them away from high jump. If they are 2 metres tall, we do not encourage them to pursue a career as a professional jockey, and so on. This takes no great foresight nor even consideration of genetic engineering. Of course these are easy examples. A more contentious one might be the use of human growth hormone for individuals who do not conform to norms for the description 'dwarfism', yet for whom additional centimetres might mean the difference between a mediocre or good sporting career and a stellar one. We have noted how Lionel Messi, one of the greatest football (soccer) players ever, benefitted precisely from this kind of intervention (Sonksen et al. 2016). The extent to which this additional height is causal to his great success is a moot point. One may also consider with some justification whether this ought to be thought of as zealous parenting, committed parenting or pediatric doping. What it does not prove is that there is a justified or widespread call for genetic engineering in order to genetically arrive at greater fairness.

How does this inform the topic at hand of genetic transfer to raise the tolerance to pain? It is undeniable that different athletes have different baselines, different capacities and different strategies to cope with pain. We do try to give people techniques to cope better with pain in everyday life, where pain management is generally not considered an essential or meaningful part of the activity we are performing. In elite-sports contexts, however, we do not give people those tools, because within certain limits tolerance to pain, as described above, is a fundamental part of practising and competing at an elite level. Pain can be distinguished from non-relevant inequalities, as for example the kind of shoes or swimsuits or bikes the athletes run, swim or cycle with, which do not impact upon the mental and physical qualities that are the source of our admiration for athletes and which are instrumental to the securing of victory. For these sorts of products, however, we can and do insist upon degrees of standardisation.

Thus, in baseball, cricket, or tennis there are regulations regarding the size and composition of the striking implement and the ball. Unusually for sports, in Formula 1 racing there is a prize for the best driver and there is a constructors' championship for the best supporting team of engineers and technologists. But even here there are strict rules about engineering variations permitted to any car. Similarly, in the Indian Premier League Cricket tournament no team can play more than four overseas players in their starting 11 in order that teams may not buy up the best global talent. Examples such as these are a commonplace. We cannot, however, 'level-out' the capacity for enduring pain in endurance events without usurping or compromising a key psychological variable inherent within the test. By levelling the ability to endure pain, we would also diminish a substantial part of the meaning of athletic performance, which can be understood as trying to break one's own limits given the starting conditions one has. That is why the toleration of pain qualifies as a relevant inequality that serves *inter alia* to demarcate athletic merit, and we consider that genetically based therapy for pain should not be permitted as it undermines the meaning of sport by interfering significantly with the relationship between natural talents, their virtuous perfection and athletic success (Murray 2009). In other words, our view of the athlete's capacity for pain tolerance could be seen as a relevant inequality and essential for the meaning of competition. Moreover, in the model developed by Loland and Hoppeler that combines a biologically based approach with a fair opportunity principle, the use of VEGF transfer could be understood as an illicit means of manipulating normal human phenotypic plasticity, and thus to go against the fair opportunity principle and the idea of the virtuous development of talent (Loland and Hoppeler 2012).

7.5 Conclusions

To sum up, the differences between the two scenarios we have presented are many and varied. We have argued that in the latter context the choice is fundamentally a self-regarding one, predicated on individual autonomy together with a risk/benefits calculation as the principal factor determining the ethics of that decision. To the contrary, in the elite endurance sports context individual autonomy ceases to play the decisive role in the ethical analysis. Sports have traditionally incorporated paternalistic practices regarding the health of competitors but also the fairness of the structuring of competition in order to produce admirable victors. The context of gene transfer matters for the evaluation of the ethical desirability or permissibility of the experimental practice we are analysing: while in an every-day-life scenario we do not accord to pain an inherently valuable role, pain does play a meaningful and constitutive role in athletic endurance competitions, along with a range of other anatomical, physiological and psychological factors. By increasing the capacity for pain tolerance, or even subtracting pain altogether from the sports experience, we would inevitably omit a fundamental part of the meaning of that picture. We conclude, therefore, that while we would not interfere with the decision of Dr House to be enrolled in a trial for VEGF-gene transfer, we could not justify the request of athletes seeking VEGF-gene transfer to increase their tolerance to pain. As a tool to cope with the intractable pain that visits afflicted patients, VEGF-gene transfer is ethically justifiable and desirable. In endurance sports, the use of VEGF-gene transfer as an endurance enhancement technology is not merely ethically unjustifiable; it compromises an element essential to the activity itself.

Notes

All websites accessed October 2017.

1 This chapter first appeared in a shorter form in *Life Sciences, Society and Policy Journal* 8(1) (2012): 20–31 with the title 'Gene Transfer for Pain: A tool to cope with the intractable, or an unethical endurance-enhancing technology?', co-authored by Camporesi and McNamee. The chapter has been substantially updated and modified. Permission to reprint is with authors, as per journal policy:

Articles in Springer Open journals do not require transfer of copyright as the copyright remains with the author. In confirming the publication of your article with open access you agree to the Creative Commons Attribution License.

2 https://clinicaltrials.gov (search performed October 2017)

3 As we write there has been considerable discussion about the IOC's dissatisfaction with the widespread systemic doping apparatus in Russia alleged prior to the 2016 Rio Olympic Games. The dispute still rumbles on with counter claims regarding the quality of evidence, and the lack of right of appeal, and so on. At present the IOC is still considering an independent testing authority for the period of the Olympic Games. Quite what 'independent' is to be understood to mean, and why it would be any more independent than WADA (who are half funded by governments and half funded by the IOC) remains unclear.

4 One notable exception is Murray (2009).

References

All websites accessed October 2017.

Baumgartner, I. 2000. Therapeutic angiogenesis: theoretic problems using vascular endothelial growth factor. *Current Cardiology Reports*, 2(1): 24–28.

Breivik, H., B. Collett, V. Ventafridda, R. Cohen and D. Gallacher. 2006. Survey of chronic pain in Europe: prevalence, impact on daily life, and treatment. *European Journal of Pain*, 10(4): 287–333.

Broglio, S.P., M. McCrea, T. McAllister, J. Harezlak, B. Katz, D. Hack, B. Hainline and CARE Consortium Investigators. 2017. A national study on the effects of concussion in collegiate athletes and US military service academy members: the NCAA–DoD Concussion Assessment, Research and Education (CARE) Consortium structure and methods. *Sports Medicine*, 47(7): 1437–1451.

Cassell, E.J. 1998. The nature of suffering and the goals of medicine. *Loss, Grief & Care*, 8(1–2): 129–142.

Crust, L. 2007. Mental toughness in sport: a review. *International Journal of Sport and Exercise Psychology*, 5(3): 270–290.

Dolgin, E. 2010. Fluctuating baseline pain implicated in failure of clinical trials. *Nature Medicine*, 16(10): 1053.

Forrest, D. and R. Simmons. 2003. Sport and gambling. *Oxford Review of Economic Policy*, 19(4): 598–611.

Freedman, B. 1987. Equipoise and the ethics of clinical research. *New England Journal of Medicine* 317(3): 141–145.

Fry, J.P. 2006. Pain, suffering and paradox in sport and religion. In *Pain and Injury in Sport: Social and Ethical Analysis*, eds S. Loland, B. Skirstad and I. Waddington. London and New York: Routledge, pp. 246–259.

Giacca, M. and S. Zacchigna. 2012. VEGF gene therapy: therapeutic angiogenesis in the clinic and beyond. *Gene Therapy*, 19(6): 622–629.

Goins, W.F., J.B. Cohen and J.C. Glorioso. 2012. Gene therapy for the treatment of chronic peripheral nervous system pain. *Neurobiology of Disease*, 48(2): 255–270.

Gucciardi, D.F., S. Gordon and J.A. Dimmock. 2009. Advancing mental toughness research and theory using personal construct psychology. *International Review of Sport and Exercise Psychology*, 2(1): 54–72.

Hämäläinen, M. 2013. Two kinds of sport records. *Sport, Ethics and Philosophy*, 7(4): 378–390.

Hamilton, T. and D. Coyle. 2013. *The Secret Race: Inside the Hidden World of the Tour de France: Doping, Cover-ups, and Winning at All Costs*. New York: Random House.

Henderson, G.E., M.M. Easter, C. Zimmer, N.M. King, A.M. Davis, B.B. Rothschild … and D.K. Nelson. 2006. Therapeutic misconception in early phase gene transfer trials. *Social Science & Medicine*, 62(1): 239–253.

Horng, S. and C. Grady. 2003. Misunderstanding in clinical research: Distinguishing therapeutic misconception, therapeutic misestimation, and therapeutic optimism. *IRB: Ethics & Human Research*, 25(1): 11–16.

Howe, P.D. 2004. *Sport, Professionalism, and Pain: Ethnographies of Injury and Risk*. London: Routledge.

Huizenga, R. 1995. *You're OK, It's Just a Bruise*. London: St Martin's Press.

Kim, H.J., S.Y. Jang, J.I. Park, J. Byun, D.I. Kim, Y.S. Do … and D.K. Kim. 2004. Vascular endothelial growth factor-induced angiogenic gene therapy in patients with peripheral artery disease. *Experimental & Molecular Medicine*, 36(4): 336–344.

Kimmelman, J. (2010). *Gene Transfer and the Ethics of First-in-human Research: Lost in Translation*. Cambridge: Cambridge University Press.

Kimmelman, J. and A. Levenstadt. 2005. Elements of style: consent form language and the therapeutic misconception in phase 1 gene transfer trials. *Human Gene Therapy*, 16(4): 502–508.

Koessler, K. 2006. Sport and the psychology of pain. In *Pain and Injury in Sport: Social and Ethical Analysis*, eds S. Loland, B. Skirstad and I. Waddington. London and New York: Routledge, pp. 34–48.

Loland, S. 2003. Fair play in sport: a moral norm system. *Sportwissenschaft*, 33(1): 90–92.

Loland, S. 2009. Fairness in sport: An ideal and its consequences. In *Performance-enhancing Technologies in Sports: Ethical, Conceptual, and Scientific Issues*, eds T.H. Murray, K.J. Maschke and A.A. Wasunna. Baltimore, MD: Johns Hopkins University Press, pp. 160–174.

Loland, S. and H. Hoppeler. (2012). Justifying anti-doping: the fair opportunity principle and the biology of performance enhancement. *European Journal of Sport Science*, 12(4): 347–353.

Loland, S. and M. McNamee. 2000. Fair play and the ethos of sports: an eclectic philosophical framework. *Journal of the Philosophy of Sport*, 27(1): 63–80.

Lurie, Y. 2006. The ontology of sports injuries and professional medical ethics. In *Pain and Injury in Sport: Social and Ethical Analysis*, eds S. Loland, B. Skirstad and I. Waddington. London and New York: Routledge, pp. 200–211.

McGrath, M. 2012. Is pain medication in sports a form of legal doping? *BBC News Science and Environment*. Available at www.bbc.co.uk/news/science-environment-18282072

McNamee, M.J. 2006. Suffering in and for sport: some philosophical remarks on a painful emotion. In *Pain and Injury in Sport: Social and Ethical Analysis*, eds S. Loland, B. Skirstad and I. Waddington. London and New York: Routledge, pp. 229–245.

McNamee, M.J. 2008. *Sports, Virtues and Vices: Morality Plays*. London: Routledge.

Mughal, N.A., D.A. Russell, S. Ponnambalam and S. Homer-Vanniasinkam. 2012. Gene therapy in the treatment of peripheral arterial disease. *British Journal of Surgery*, 99(1): 6–15.

Munting, R. 1996. *An Economic and Social History of Gambling*. Manchester: Manchester University Press.

Muona, K., K. Mäkinen, M. Hedman, H. Manninen and S. Ylä-Herttuala. 2012. 10-year safety follow-up in patients with local VEGF gene transfer to ischemic lower limb. *Gene Therapy*, 19(4), 392–395.

Murray, T.H. 2009. Ethics and endurance-enhancing technologies in sport. In *Performance-enhancing Technologies in Sports: Ethical, Conceptual, and Scientific Issues*, eds T.H. Murray, K.J. Maschke and A.A. Wasunna. Baltimore, MD: Johns Hopkins University Press, pp. 141–159.

Nixon, H.L. 1992. A social network analysis of influences on athletes to play with pain and injuries. *Journal of Sport and Social Issues*, 16(2): 127–135.

Nixon, H.L. 1993. Accepting the risks of pain and injury in sport: mediated cultural influences on playing hurt. *Sociology of Sport Journal*, 10(2): 183–196.

Schubert, M. and T. Könecke. 2015. 'Classical' doping, financial doping and beyond: UEFA's financial fair play as a policy of anti-doping. *International Journal of Sport Policy and Politics*, 7(1): 63–86.

Sonksen, P.H., D. Cowan and R. Holt. 2016. Use and misuse of hormones in sport. *The Lancet Diabetes and Endocrinology*: 882–883.

Springer, M.L., A.S. Chen, P.E. Kraft, M. Bednarski and H.M. Blau. 1998. VEGF gene delivery to muscle: potential role for vasculogenesis in adults. *Molecular Cell*, 2(5): 549–558.

Tännsjö, T. 2010. Medical enhancement and the ethos of elite sport. In *Human Enhancement*, eds J. Savulescu and N. Bostrom. Oxford: Oxford University Press, pp. 315–326.

Tracey, I. and M.C. Bushnell. 2009. How neuroimaging studies have challenged us to rethink: Is chronic pain a disease? *The Journal of Pain*, 10(11): 1113–1120.

WADA [World Anti-Doping Agency]. 2015. *World Anti-Doping Code*. Available at: www.wada-ama.org/en/resources/the-code/world-anti-doping-code

8

ON THE ELIGIBILITY OF FEMALE ATHLETES WITH HYPERANDROGENISM TO COMPETE: ATHLETICISM, MEDICALISATION AND TESTOSTERONE

8.1 Introduction[1]

While this is not a work of feminist scholarship *per se*, one cannot help but align oneself with feminists when considering the history of sport. It has been, and continues to be, a male domain. As historian of medicine and sport Vanessa Heggie writes: 'Women and girls had, of course, already been identified as abnormal by other medical professionals, and their exclusion from physical activity was part of a larger, non-sport specific construction of their physiology' (Heggie 2011, 16). In many countries the tensions between perceived femininity and athleticism still haunt women's participation in sport (Schneider 2000). And while, in the Western world, equality of opportunity exists in public funding of sport, this is a fairly low benchmark. Other achievements, such as the Title IX legislation in the USA regarding non-discrimination on the grounds of sex in educational institutions, have brought about huge advances in women's sports in terms of equal funding for programmes, coaching support and so on, at least in theory. Clearly the times have been changing for some decades and though battles have been won the 'war' is far from over.

Notwithstanding legal and soft policy towards respect and proper treatment of a range of gender-driven problems, there is one class of athletes whose gender has signalled great problems not merely on a cultural or social level, but also – and powerfully – on a biological and especially genetic level. In this chapter we discuss two recent important cases in elite sport in which the female body has been constructed as 'other' or 'abnormal', namely the bodies of South African middle-distance runner Caster Semenya and of Indian sprinter Dutee Chand. We first present Semenya's case, which triggered the drafting of the 2011 International Association of Athletics Federations (IAAF: the international governing body regulating athletics competition worldwide) regulations on eligibility of female athletes with hyperandrogenism to compete in the female category (hence, 'Hyperandrogenism

Regulations'). We then critically analyse the IAAF regulations both from a scientific and from an ethical point of view, before discussing Dutee Chand's case and her appeal to the Court of Arbitration for Sport (CAS: the international body that settles sports disputes worldwide). In the second part of this chapter we comment on the CAS landmark decision (July 2015) to suspend the regulations for two years pending further evidence from the IAAF, and the more recent developments of the case (July 2017). We conclude by commenting on other ethically problematic issues pertaining to women's competition in elite sport.

8.2 Caster Semenya's case

Caster Semenya, the multiple-medal-winning South African middle-distance runner, is only one case in a long line of women athletes who have fallen foul of zealous (typically male) sports regulators and institutional bodies ever since the Federation Sportive Feminine International persuaded the International Olympic Committee (IOC) to permit five women's track and field events in the 1928 Olympic Games in Amsterdam (Schultz 2012). By 1936 the controversial conservative US President of the IOC, Avery Brundage, had stipulated that 'all women athletes entered into the Olympics be subjected to a thorough physical examination to make sure they were really 100% female' (ibid., 106). The Cold War exacerbated these problems with Western journalists, athletes and administrators routinely complaining about the masculinisation of female athletes. Physical observation to determine sex status continued until the late 1960s. Mary Peters, later to win the gold in pentathlon in 1972 for Great Britain and Northern Ireland, wrote graphically of a manual internal gynecological examination that was tantamount to groping (ibid.). It was not until 1967 that the IAAF developed and administered a laboratory-based chromosomal test, avoiding some (though not all) of the indignity of the previous regimes' practices.

As it is presently structured, much of sport is predicated on a range of criteria that build classes of categories of competition. Gender, for historical reasons, has been the most prominent, though its foundational reason of 'equality of opportunity' is far from obvious in many cases. Hence the *prima facie* need for some form of discrimination among the participants who appear to blur preconceptions of male/female stereotypes. The process was known as gender verification (Skirstad 2000), an especially ironic descriptor since as Daniels (1992) argues, gender is a social construct and no biological test can verify that. Evidently the test is aimed at distinguishing among biological sexes, male and female. Moreover, proof positive, in the form of a certificate, was usually required for eligibility purposes. The Spanish athlete Martínez-Patiño tells the harrowing story of forgetting her certificate at the 1985 World University Games in Kobe, Japan only to be tested anew with a further test and be disqualified from the competition (Martínez-Patiño 2005).

Fifty years of 'gender verification' have focused on the 'Three Gs: genitals, gonads, and genetic material' (Schultz 2012, 32). The IAAF has worked through a series of reforms in an attempt to cater for the complex mélange of ethical issues, but it is certainly the case of Caster Semenya that brought the matter to a head, and which has brought about the IAAF's most sophisticated guidelines to date (Montañola and Olivesi 2016).

Caster Semenya competed at the Berlin IAAF Track Championship in 2009, where she won the 800 metres with 1:56.72, two and a half seconds ahead of the runner-up. Only a few hours after the end of the race, the IAAF revoked her medal and started an investigation regarding her 'gender' eligibility. The IAAF reported that the 'incredible improvement in the athlete's performance' triggered the investigation and compared her improvement to 'the sort of dramatic break-throughs that usually arouse suspicion of drug abuse' (Camporesi and Maugeri 2010). The IAAF banned Semenya from competitions during the investigations. Semenya was eventually reinstated to compete after an 11-month investigation, but the results of her tests were never made public.

It is important to note that in 2009 there were no guidelines regulating 'gender' testing, as the IAAF had abandoned all testing in 1991, and the IOC had also done so in 1999 (Elsas et al. 2000). As reported by Heggie (2010, 7), the IAAF argued that gender testing was no longer necessary because 'modern sportswear was now so revealing that it seemed unfeasible that a man could masquerade as a woman', which had been the main concern underlying the gender testing regulations. After concerns for false positive results at the Atlanta Olympic Games in 1996, in 1999 the IOC also removed the requirements for gender testing.

In the case of sex differentiation a broad spectrum of conditions lies between the two categories 'male' and 'female'. As a matter of fact, the number of deviations from statistically normal traits – often referred with the medicalised term 'disorders of sex differentiation' – can be counted in the order of tens and can be classified as sex chromosome, gonadal and sex hormone deviations (or abnormalities if we want to stick to the medical terminology) (Yang et al. 2010). About 1.7% of people has one of these conditions. Only some of these are apparent, and many people who have them do not discover they belong to this 1.7% until they decide to have children and find out that they are subfertile or sterile. For the sake of illustration, people with complete androgen insensitivity syndrome (CAIS) are genetically XY (chromosomally, males), have testes and testosterone levels in the normal range of the male population. Nevertheless, these individuals have a thoroughly feminine phenotype, with breast and female typical genitalia, because they are unable to metabolise androgens. If we take their genetic make-up into account, these individuals would be classified as males. Nevertheless, their metabolic levels of androgens are in the standard female range and they overwhelmingly identify, and are identified, as women. These examples show already how great human physical variance is, and how difficult it is to force such a variety into rigidly binary ontologies.

Semenya's case triggered the IAAF, in coordination with the IOC, to revisit the guidelines for when a woman should be allowed to compete as a woman. The *IAAF Regulations Governing Eligibility of Females with Hyperandrogenism to Compete in Women's Competition* came into force in May 2011, shortly followed by similar IOC policies.[2] Although neither IAAF nor IOC mention explicitly a relation between

Caster Semenya and the regulations, this is quite apparent and an extensive body of critical literature has been written on the subject (Cooky et al. 2013; Montañola and Olivesi 2016; Schultz 2012; Teetzel 2014).

8.3 The Hyperandrogenism Regulations

Hyperandrogenism is a medical condition defined as 'a state characterized or caused by an excessive secretion of androgens by the adrenal cortex, ovaries, or testes'.[3] The term is most commonly used in reference to women, against whom there is a norm of what should count as 'excessive' level of androgens (see below for a discussion of this norm). One of the most common causes of hyperandrogenism is polycystic ovaric syndrome, which is an endocrine condition affecting up to 15–20% of women of reproductive age, where ovaries contain multiple follicles which lead to irregular menstrual periods and can lead to excess acne, excess hair and in more severe and rare cases to a number of co-morbidities including metabolic syndrome, hypertension, dyslipidemia, glucose intolerance and diabetes. Other less common (and less benign) causes of hyperandrogenism can be ovarian tumours or tumours of adrenal glands (Sirmans and Pate 2014; Housman and Reynolds 2014). It is important to note that hyperandrogenism does not pose an immediate threat to the health of the person affected, and is generally not medicated except in very severe cases, to prevent the insurgence of co-morbidities, as we discuss at length below.

The 2011 Hyperandrogenism Regulations require female athletes who do not fall within the limits of 100 ng/dL2 of testosterone to undergo androgen-suppressive therapy for up to two years in order to reduce the level of testosterone and compete as females. In other words, women with endogenous levels of testosterone (endogenous meaning produced naturally by their bodies, in contrast to the external administration of testosterone through pharmaceuticals or gene transfer) are considered to have an 'excess' level of testosterone.

The 'unfair advantage' thesis is the assumption underlying IAAF regulations on hyperandrogenism. Paragraph 6.5 of the IAAF policies on eligibility of women with hyperandrogenism to compete in women's competition states this quite clearly:

> The Expert Medical Panel shall recommend that the athlete is eligible to compete in women's competition if:
>
> i   she has androgen levels below the normal male range; or
> ii she has androgen levels within the normal male range but has an androgen resistance such that she derives no competitive advantage from having androgen levels in the normal male range.[4]

The assumption has historically been that hyperandrogenism leads inexorably to inequality in sports contests that are women-only. Moreover, it is considered that the inequality represents an unmerited advantage for the athlete who has the condition. In a move of hard paternalism, the IAAF requires that the athletes submit themselves to a pharmacological intervention that can be seen as a coercive offer. Since there is no sport philosophical literature here to guide the aptness of this description, and the bioethical literature aligns typically to the delivery of a medical service or good, we refer to the conditions laid out by Lyons (1975, 436) as a template:

1. P knows that Q is rationally reluctant to give y to P for x; and
2. Either Q knows that [s]he has a right to x from P on easier terms, or Q knows that P would have given x to Q, on easier terms, if the chance had not arisen to trade x for y.

The model is not perfect as a precedent. We thus interpret it as follows: if an athlete wants to continue as an athlete in races governed by IAAF (i.e. all elite athlete events), the Hyperandrogenism Regulations must be accepted. Thus Semenya, and others like her (P), have dedicatedly trained for years to achieve elite status; they clearly have a strong identification with the activity, and it is likely to be their main source of economic livelihood. They believe they are entitled to participate. The IAAF (Q) knows that athletes with genetic abnormalities are not normally prevented from participation on those grounds, but are in a monopolistic position to demand a pharmacological protocol in order to permit participation (thus the athlete must trade acceptance of the protocol for eligibility).

As noted, the IAAF and IOC policies require female athletes who do not fall within the limits of 100 ng/dL2 of testosterone to undergo androgen-suppressive therapy for up to two years in order to reduce the level of testosterone and be eligible to compete as females. The test is not one of sex *per se*, but a biomarker proxy used to determine eligibility. According to the IAAF/IOC, mandated pharmacological treatment reduces testosterone in order to restore the level playing field. This in effect is to alter natural inequalities that they believe threaten the sex-segregated integrity of competition.

The requirement to undergo medical treatment put forward by the IAAF/IOC is of course highly disrespectful of the autonomy of the individuals involved – although it is reasonable to speculate that, when required (i.e. as a coercive offer), athletes are likely to comply with the intervention. Nevertheless, it is important to recall that in biomedical ethics the principle of 'respect for autonomy' cannot be reduced to 'compliance under the threat of a sanction' (i.e. non-participation). Indeed, there are good reasons to think that the 'consent' (such as it is) obtained in the circumstances here reviewed will be invalid. In this context, the potential for coercion is more than an academic hypothesis, as athletes are, more or less explicitly, asked to choose whether to end their professional careers or to submit to an intervention they have no desire to undertake (Camporesi and Maugeri 2016). Nor it is clear that we can properly describe this as a treatment since it is neither desired by the athlete-patient, nor necessarily indicative of a pathology. Based on these grounds, it seems that the intervention is a sporting one, not a medical one.

It is suggested (Pierson 2011) that previous gender verification tests were more about identifying hormonal manipulation than uncovering genetic abnormalities and attempting to preserve athletic competition classes. Nevertheless, in the case of hyperandrogenism (and related disorders) the IAAF may well have wisely attempted to avoid the profound ontological questions concerning 'womanhood' (a question they specifically set aside with the abandonment of all gender testing policies in 1999), and assumed an easier route via the Hyperandrogenism Regulations. Their focus is now on ethically justifiable eligibility: when womanhood and fair competition are coexistent. This leaves us with the deceptively simple philosophical question: what is it that makes a 'woman' (and *mutatis mutandis* 'man') for the purposes of sports competitions? Or what constitutes a 'sportswoman' or 'sportsman'?

8.4 Inconclusive evidence

One obvious answer is also deceptively simple: testosterone. As we read in the regulations, 'The difference in athletic performance between males and females is known to be predominantly due to higher levels of androgenic hormones in males resulting in increased strength and muscle development'. Testosterone, hence, becomes the master molecule of 'athleticism' and, more importantly for our purposes, the biochemical watershed of 'masculinity' and 'femininity'.

The idea that an extremely complex trait like athleticism can be reduced to one single biochemical component, to a 'master molecule of athleticism', and in a way that markedly discriminates between 'males' and 'females', is wholly problematic. As shown by Karkazis and Jordan-Young (2013), it is not precisely clear how testosterone works with regard to athleticism, but what is clear is that testosterone cannot be used to predict who is going to perform better, nor it can be used to infer that people who perform better have more testosterone. Testosterone is portrayed as a 'male' molecule and its effects are said to confer 'masculine traits', yet testosterone is of course also found in women's bodies. In the literature on sex-determination femaleness is always conceptualised in terms of the absence of a male-determining factor, or the presence of the passive form of that factor. More-over, although the reference range for testosterone for adult males is comprised between 300 and 1200 ng/dL and for adult females it does not exceed, on average, 100 ng/dL, it has been observed that testosterone concentrations vary according to several factors such as exposure to exogenous hormones such as estrogen and thyroxine, diurnal variation and the age of the individual (Bostwick and Joyner 2012).

As we will discuss below, the July 2015 suspension of the regulations following Dutee Chand's appeal to the Court of Arbitration for Sport in Lausanne is grounded exactly on the point that the IAAF has not sufficiently proven that testosterone confers an advantage in competition. However, as we argue in the remainder of this chapter, even if that were the case, such an advantage would not necessarily be unfair. This calls the IAAF regulations seriously into question.

Moving from a medical to a sport-ethical standpoint, it is important to highlight the auxiliary assumptions that seemingly prompted the classificatory effort within the regulations. Indeed, in the IAAF regulations on hyperandrogenism, classificatory efforts coalesce with normative concerns about fairness in sports, in an attempt to preserve the idea of the level playing field. The moral and political concept of 'fairness' and its metaphorical operationalisation of 'level playing field' appear to be the fundamental normative drivers of the issue. It is thus necessary to spell out whether cases of hyperandrogenism would actually challenge them in an ethically relevant way. Let us therefore take as a premise of our arguments the assumption that higher levels of testosterone *do* confer an athletic advantage. We argue below that, even based on this premise, the medicalisation of athletes with hyperandrogenism is unwarranted, as it ultimately results in inconsistent policies and, more importantly, in markedly discriminatory attitudes towards athletes' improperly pathologised bodies.

8.5 Unfair advantage? Inconsistencies in the regulations

In a response letter to Karkazis and co-authors (2012) published in *The American Journal of Bioethics*, the authors of the IAAF Hyperandrogenism Regulations – while recognising that drawing a line on such a complex continuum is controversial – defend the policy, arguing that it responds sufficiently well to the 'limited purpose of providing for fair competition in sport' with regard to possible cases of hyperandrogenism (Bermon et al. 2013). Along similar lines, Eric Vilain (medical geneticist at UCLA and member of the IOC Medical Commission) has argued that, while imperfect, the policies represent an improvement on what we had before (Macur 2014). This latter point may well be the case, but it is not clear that this is sufficient warrant to coerce athletes into a programme of pharmacological testosterone depletion.

Bermon and co-authors argue that the Hyperandrogenism Regulations, although bound to be controversial, are 'a vast improvement over previous efforts' and 'respond with sensitivity to possible cases of hyperandrogenisation' in that the new policies represent 'fairness for female athletes, respect for all' (Bermon et al. 2013). Somewhat surprisingly, however, they make no attempt to try to distinguish between advantage and unfair advantage. Rather, they write:

> The female former Olympic athletes, who contributed to the creation of the IAAF regulations, agreed that success in sport should be due to the combination of talent and dedication. In events where androgenisation provides a powerful advantage, women want to compete against alike, not against women with a degree of hyperandrogenism that gives them a male physiology.
>
> *(Bermon et al. 2013, 65)*

In the present case we could say that Caster Semenya may have had a property advantage (following Hämäläinen 2012, discussed in Chapter 5), defined as the level of testosterone. We say 'may', since in protecting her right to medical confidentiality, we do not know for a fact which condition she is affected by.

Nevertheless, even if this were the case, this would be only one of the factors that contributed to her superior athletic performance at the 2009 World Championships 800 metres final in Berlin. More importantly, it does not follow from the fact that she may have a property advantage, that this property advantage would be unfair to her fellow athletes in competition.

The very notion of a level playing field is a piece of folk psychology. Everyone knows that it is a metaphor and that metaphors ought not to be pressed into serious policy and practice. The level playing field metaphor serves as a useful heuristic. It is impossible to level out all inequalities. And by the very logic of sport we are fascinated by how contests can reveal athletic inequalities in order to evaluate, compare, rank and so on (Loland 2002). The long-standing moral imperative ruling of fairness in sports, or fair opportunity as Loland and Hoppeler (2012) have argued, becomes the essence of ethical concerns in the IAAF Regulations. The regulatory normativity, as we have seen above, acknowledges – and indeed is motivated by – the need to accommodate borderline cases (i.e. instances of hyperandrogenism). The accommodation of cases that fail to conform to the standard, however, comes about through the pathologisation of transgressive bodies. If you want to be a woman, one that is fair to her fellow competitors, you must have the right level of androgens either by 'nature' or after submitting to medical treatment (Camporesi and Maugeri 2016).

Why are the IAAF and IOC targeting only hyperandrogenism among the many genetic and biological variations that provide a property advantage? Why do they not consider unfair all the other genetic and biological variations that confer a performance advantage? We think that the answer can only lie in the following: hyperandrogenism gets singled out from all other biological and genetic variations as it challenges deeply entrenched social beliefs concerning the dominant stereotype of femininity in a way that other variations do not.

8.6 Perception as trigger for testing and the burden of performing femininity on track and field

'These kind of people should not run with us. For me, she is not a woman. She's a man' (Clarey and Kolata 2009). This is what Elisa Cusma, a disappointed Italian runner who finished sixth, was reported saying about Caster Semenya's victory in the 800 metres final of the 2009 Berlin World Athletics Championships. In Elisa Cusma's words we find encapsulated the reasons that have long supported sex segregation in sports competitions. We also find encapsulated the link with women athletes' bodily transformations and appearances: a woman in sport should look like a woman, according to the IAAF and IOC, where 'visual perception' becomes the trigger for testing.

Of course perceptions need not be accurate nor fair. Cooky and Dworkin (2013) highlight the mis/appropriation of racist and nationalist narratives to defend Semenya's sexual identity. Fabien Rose (2016) describes how merely the perception of sexual otherness explicitly becomes an appropriate tool of detection for 'sex'.

Women who do not conform to heteronormative (and Western) standards of femininity, such as Caster Semenya, become targets for others' perceptions, which in turn trigger investigations. This assumption is illustrated by a table produced in appendix 2 of the IAAF policies,[5] showing various signs of 'virilization' on various body parts (upper lip, chin, chest, abdomen, arms, thigh and back), which are supposed to constitute many traces of hormonal nonconformity. As pointed out by Roger J. Pielke, the language of the IOC has not changed much in the past 40 years (Pielke 2016). Writing in 1974, Eduardo Hay of the IOC Medical Commission provided a window into the thinking behind the policies of that era: 'Today the purpose of the femininity tests carried out on women athletes taking part in the Olympic Games is to make sure that all female athletes compete under identical anatomical conditions' (Hay 1974). Titled 'Hirsutism scoring sheet according to Ferriman and Gallwey', this scoring sheet identifies nine 'clinical signs' used to identify possible hyperandrogenism in female athletes. Hence, while the IAAF no longer uses the term 'femininity' in its regulations, it nonetheless displays a marked focus on what are broadly considered to be 'feminine' physical characteristics, such as (lack of) body hair and the size and shape of breasts. Visual cues become a 'trigger' for testing. Sports therefore become the new arena for the re-enactment of traditional gender performances, as argued by Judith Butler (1990). Examples of gender performativity in track and field abound. Think for example of American sprinter 'Flo-Jo' (Florence Griffith Joyner), who used to run with very long painted nails, or more recently of Russian pole-vaulter Elena Isinbayeva, another emblem of femininity in track and field, or of American athlete Maggie Wessey, who used to run the 800 metres with Nike's hyper-feminised outfits (Camporesi 2017).

8.7 Unnecessary medicalisation and burden of cost on athletes

There seem to be at least two additional layers of analysis that need unpacking: (a) issues with the medicalisation of healthy bodies in order to compete; (b) questions of reinforcement of systemic disadvantages, as the costs for the medical interventions recommended by the policies fall on the athletes.

In accordance with established principles of medical ethics, medical interventions are to be administered only if they are for the benefit of the patients and are done in a manner respectful of their autonomy. Ruling that people with higher-than-the-norm levels of androgens are eligible to compete only after submitting to a medical test violates both principles. On the one hand, hyperandrogenism does not – in most cases – pose an immediate threat to the health of the person affected. As discussed above, medical evidence shows that high level of androgens only increase the risk of hirsutism, acne, possibly alopecia and have other virilising cutaneous manifestations (Housman and Reynolds 2014); but none of these augmented risks is incompatible with physical activity or participation in elite sport. There are many women out there affected by hyperandrogenism (polycystic ovaric syndrome is one of the more common conditions that causes it, with a prevalence of between 10 and 15% of all women), but they do not have to take androgen suppressive therapy or undergo surgeries.

As reported by Fénichel and co-authors, four unnamed female athletes were found to have levels of androgens outside the 'normal' female range set by the IAAF/IOC (Fénichel et al. 2013). They were all subjected to unnecessary medicalisation procedures that had nothing to do with reducing testosterone levels in sport, including vaginoplasty and partial cliteridectomy. Fénichel and co-authors have argued – rightly, in our opinion – that the additional feminising procedures are 'particularly alarming', and the notion that the policies emanate out of a 'concern for the health of the athletes' (cf. Bermon et al. 2013) is unwarranted. This assertion ignores the fact that the women may not want the interventions, especially if they are not medically necessary but are only necessary conditions to re-enter the field of play. Equally, they may feel they have no non-coercive choice.

Laurence Brunet and Muriel Salle (2016) offer a unique comparative historical overview of the legal panorama for intersex people, and show that society is moving towards laws that prohibit surgeries on children to fix disorders of sex development. The first example of this law in Europe was promulgated in Malta in 2015, banning sex reassignment surgeries or treatment on minors on the basis that they lack medical justification and can be postponed until the child is old enough to assert informed consent. Another decisive step in this direction has been the adoption in 2013 by the Parliamentary Assembly of the Council of Europe of a resolution devoted to the right of intersex children to physical integrity,[6] which goes hand in hand with an explicit condemnation of medical and surgical treatments imposed on children when they are not vital to the child's health.

It seems, however, that the world of competitive sports is surprisingly detached from these recent progressive legal developments by requiring women to have to undergo androgen suppressive therapies or other sexual 'normalisation' surgeries in order to compete which are increasingly discouraged or banned worldwide. From this perspective the policies of the IAAF and IOC are, to say the least, anachronistic.

Finally, it is important to note that while the policies explicitly recommend treatment, they also explicitly state that they will not cover the costs for medical intervention (paragraph 7.4 of the IAAF 2011 regulations).[7] Nor, we may assume, will they cover the costs of genetic and other counselling to enable athletes to understand properly the conditions they have and the implications of treatment or non-treatment decisions. In other words, not only is the burden of proof to demonstrate androgen resistance on the athlete (paragraph 6.6 of the rules),[8] but so is the 'burden of cost' for the interventions against hyperandrogenism that is the required procedure to get them back to the track. It goes without saying that athletes like Caster Semenya, who grew up in the village of Limpopo in rural north-western South Africa, in the 'middle of nowhere' according to the people of South Africa, as reported in Levy (2009), or Dutee Chand, daughter of weavers who make $8 a week, as reported in Macur (2014), are seriously disadvantaged by the sex test policies. We now turn to Dutee Chand's case.

8.8 Dutee Chand, the suspension of the regulations and its implications for hyperandrogenic athletes

Dutee Chand is a promising Indian sprinter. Born in 1996, in 2012 she became a national champion in the under-18 category in the 100 metres event, but was disqualified just days before the beginning of the 2014 Commonwealth Games in Glasgow after a medical test determined that her levels of testosterone were above the 10 nmol/ Lit limit set by the IAAF Hyperandrogenism Regulations. According to IAAF regulations, if Chand were able to reduce her androgen levels she would be allowed to resume competition. Chand refused to do so and appealed to the Court of Arbitration for Sport (CAS), with the financial support from the sports ministry of India.[9] Her appeal took place at CAS headquarters in Lausanne, Switzerland, on 26–28 March 2015.

On 27 July 2015, the CAS announced that the Hyperandrogenism Regulations would be suspended for the next two years in order to give the IAAF the opportunity to provide the CAS with scientific evidence about the quantitative relationship between enhanced testosterone levels and improved athletic performance in hyperandrogenic athletes. If the IAAF is unable to produce such evidence, the regulations will be considered void. Indeed, the CAS panel has concluded that there is 'presently insufficient evidence about the degree of advantage that androgen-sensitive hyperandrogenic females enjoy over non-hyperandrogenic females',[10] and has asked the IAAF to demonstrate a 'correlation' between levels of testosterone in female athletes and competitive advantage. So the CAS has requested proof that there is indeed an advantage derived from higher levels of testosterone. While the suspension of the regulations was clearly reason to rejoice in the short term for Dutee Chand and for other athletes with hyperandrogenism, who were allowed to resume competition, it was concerning that the proviso for the suspension of the regulations fell within the scientific track of the IAAF, as noted by Camporesi of the authors shortly after the CAS interim award (Camporesi 2016).

The CAS panel explicitly stated that the IAAF assumption (that increased testosterone confers an advantage) 'may well be proved valid' (paragraph 543), but concluded that sufficient evidence had not been provided to show evidence of correlation, and that the 'onus of proof' remained on the IAAF (paragraph 534). The CAS panel has suggested a suspension of the Hyperandrogenism Regulations for a maximum period of two years in order to give the IAAF the opportunity to provide the CAS with additional scientific evidence about the quantitative relationship between enhanced testosterone levels and improved athletic performance in hyperandrogenic athletes. In other words, the CAS is aligned to the view that if testosterone is proven to give an athletic advantage, then the regulations should be reinstated. Indeed, the IAAF was quick to note that the CAS panel's ruling stated there is '*a sound scientific basis to the Regulations*' [emphasis added] in that endogenous testosterone is 'the best indicator of performance differences between male and female athletes', and that the court accepted that hyperandrogenic female athletes may have a competitive advantage over athletes with testosterone levels in the normal female range (IAAF 2015).

Nevertheless, as we have argued above, adopting such a line of argumentation is grounded in both normative and scientific assumptions rather than in something more approaching certainty. That is, even if testosterone did confer an athletic advantage that could be proven by the IAAF upon submission of further evidence, this advantage would not be unfair. Hence, even if the IAAF were able to prove that there is a correlation between higher levels of testosterone and a competitive advantage, this would not constitute sufficient grounds for the reinstatement of the regulations. In anticipation of Semenya's victory at the 2016 Rio Olympic Games, the controversy around her supposed 'unfair advantage' in competition was fuelled by the media, who must bear some responsibility in her maltreatment. In a feature article, the *Guardian* referred to her participation in Rio as a 'ticking time bomb'.[11] South African sport scientist Ross Tucker – who disagreed with the suspension of the regulations – also suggested that a good performance by Semenya provided the IAAF with a reason to go back to the court and say 'here you go – here's your evidence'. And this is exactly what happened. Shortly after Semenya's victory in Rio, Lord Sebastian Coe, former British middle-distance Olympic champion, chief organiser of the London 2012 Olympics and current president of IAAF, announced that IAAF would bring in more evidence to the CAS to re-open the case.[12] While the IAAF was initially granted two years (until the end of July 2017) to submit additional evidence to initiate an appeal, on 28 July 2017 the CAS granted the IAAF two extra additional months to submit the requested additional evidence (Harper 2017; *Hindustan Times* 2017).

An article authored by Bermon and Garnier (one of the signatories of the original Hyperandrogenism Regulations in 2011), and published in the *British Journal of Sport Medicine* in early July 2017 (Bermon and Garnier 2017) reports an association between higher levels of serum androgens (i.e. levels of testosterone in the blood) and increased athletic performance in five track and field events (400m, 400m hurdles, 800m, hammer throw and pole vault). In particular, the authors argue that women with higher levels of testosterone in their blood obtain a benefit on athletic performance of between 1.8 and 4.5% compared to women with lower levels of testosterone. The results of the article have already been hailed by the press as evidence to justify a reinstatement of hyperandrogenism regulations (IAAF appeal to CAS), at least for a limited number of track & field events (Harper 2017).

However, it should be noted that such conclusions are – to say the least – premature, as the results of the study do not demonstrate the benefit of endogenous testosterone levels on athletic performance, because the data are not cross-validated with the results of athletic events. The authors only assume that a higher level of testosterone corresponds with a higher athletic performance. As put by the authors, 'Our study design cannot provide evidence for causality between androgen levels and athletic performance, but can indicate associations between androgen concentrations and athletic performance' (Bermon and Garnier 2017, 2).

In addition, the article does not distinguish between the different causes of hyperandrogenism, as the data collected do not distinguish between endogenous and exogenous causes (something which was explicitly requested by the 2015 CAS interim award):

> We deliberately decided not to exclude performances achieved by females with biological hyperandrogenism and males with biological hypoandrogenism whatever the cause of their condition (oral contraceptives, polycystic ovaries syndrome, disorder of sex development, doping, overtraining).
>
> *(Bermon and Garnier 2017, 2)*

Hence, the article does not answer the CAS' explicit requirement of scientific evidence regarding the athletic performance of athletes with hyperandrogenism which could be compared with the difference in performance which exists between men and women (10–12%), to be demonstrated with levels of endogenous testosterone.

Instead, the conclusions of the article refer to five events (400m, 400m hurdles, 800m, hammer throw and pole vault) in which women with higher levels of testosterone obtain a benefit on athletic performance of 1.8–4.5 %, which is not even close to the reported benefit required from CAS (10–12%), to demonstrate a difference in performance between women with hyperandrogenism and women without. In addition, if we take into account that in the study 21 events were analysed, only five of which demonstrated a benefit from testosterone levels on athletic performance, this amounts to a mere 23.8% of the total number of events analysed. That seems like straight cherry-picking of results.[13]

This said, the arguments of this chapter would still be valid even if there were clear evidence that endogenous testosterone had a definite impact on athletic performance. This is because the answer to the question of whether women with hyperandrogenism should be allowed to compete in the female category is not to be found in data showing that (and to what extent) testosterone confers an advantage in competition. In other words, the question should not be: will more research prove the correlation between increased testosterone levels and athletic performance? Instead, we should ask ourselves the question: what are we trying to prove when we ask for more research? As we highlighted at the beginning of this chapter, questions regarding when it is fair for a woman with hyperandrogenism to compete in the female category cannot be found either in the results of a scientific study, or of a medical evaluation. Instead, they should be found in the answer to the question: what counts as fairness in competition? A wrong question leads necessarily to a wrong answer.

To reiterate an important point made earlier in this chapter, there is no level playing field in elite sport and testosterone is no different from other advantages (e.g. body size, genetic and biological variations …) that we see at the Olympics. Think of American swimmers Ledecky and Phelps, who have dominated respectively the last Olympics in Rio and the London and Beijing Olympics. Think of American gymnast Simone Biles, who has won several medals at the 2016 Rio Olympics. Is it unfair for fellow athletes to compete in the same category as these athletes, who obviously seem to fall in a separate league? The way in which humans group things is not merely a reading of an alleged 'natural order', rather it is a more complex social activity requiring negotiation and reflection upon the consequences and the purposes of such an ordering. Moreover, there are sports where external modifications are made to redress advantages. These might include adding weights, such as happens in horse racing. Might one not consider weighted clothing? Could one also consider modifying the track – 200m and 400m runners start at different positions around the bend, and these could be modified at the highest level of competition with a temporary start position. Many such improvisations might be considered, and be more respectful of the athlete's genetically acquired biology. Of course, implementing such modifications would be difficult to achieve without stigmatising them at the same time. To coerce the athlete to undertake unwarranted medically supervised testosterone depletions is an assault on their dignity.

In a similar mode, Sherwin and Schwartz (2005, 20) argue against Tännsjö and Tamburrini's argument that the genetic enhancement of women is desirable in order that they might become 'Bio-Amazons' and thus have equality to compete on a level playing field with men. They write:

> Requiring oppressed groups to be the same as dominant groups in order to be given equal respect creates a double-bind because the group is usually oppressed on the very basis of some difference, e.g., gender, skin color, sexual orientation, or (dis)ability. Basing equality on the presumption of sameness is likely to disadvantage these people by denying the reality and implications of their difference. Since some of these differences are important to the person's identity and self-conception, and others are beyond their power to change, the suggestion that they need to assimilate to the norm that arose in their absence based on standards appropriate to the dominant group may be both impossible and offensive.

While no attempt is being made here to suggest a translation from hyperandrogenic females being forced to compete with males, there is something of this kind of coercion going on in our pharmacological normalising of the hyperandrogenic female. What seems improper is the scientifically conceived normalisation – as if that were some normatively uncontentious scientific procedure, which denies the hyperandrogenic athlete's sense of identity and self-respect. In both cases we suggested that the biological manipulation is an assault on the very dignity of the women under consideration.

By looking at the whole Semenya debacle from this perspective, it is not hard to recognise that the medicalised discourse of the IAAF and IOC apparently runs counter to the very same principle of fair play that the policies purport to protect. In other words, the policies deprive female athletes of the essence of athletic performance, which, borrowing from Murray, is both a 'celebration of and a challenge posed by our embodiment' (Murray 2009, 236). By doing so, they 'dis-embody' female athletes in competition and they not only fail to achieve the ideal of fairness they aim for; they also deprive female athletes with hyperandrogenism of the essence of sport, i.e. of the possibility of pushing their bodies to their limits thanks to an unpredictable combination of biology, talent and dedication.

8.9 Conclusions

The IAAF and IOC policies locate the process of eligibility to compete within a discourse of fair play that is itself situated within a medicalised conceptualisation of sex. As we argued elsewhere, answers as to who should be eligible to compete in which category are not to be found in allegedly unambiguous readings of 'nature' through the lenses of science or medicine. They require, instead, a broader reflection on the value and the meaning of sport: what kind of activity it is, what is the meaning of athletic excellence and why we cherish it so much. It is this kind of analysis (or its lack thereof) that, ultimately, proves the aftermath of Caster Semenya's and Dutee Chand's cases to be disconcerting.

As we have shown in this chapter, narratives of medical reductionism and of a mythical level playing field reinforce each other. IAAF and IOC regulations are permeated by outdated discourses of a binary switch of sex determination (i.e. male or female) and by the quest for a clear and precisely measurable dividing line where there is none. Questions pertaining to the construction of categories in sport cannot be found solely in science, but we keep looking for new biomedical findings that support this, although after decades of gender testing we should really know better (Shani and Barilan 2012).

As we have shown, the world of competitive sports is also alarmingly detached from recent progressive legal developments in requiring women to have to undergo androgen suppressive therapies or other sexual 'normalisation' surgeries in order to compete, which are increasingly discouraged or banned in other contexts worldwide. From this point of view the world of competitive sports is still living in the past century, and is detached from progressive laws that condemn medical and surgical treatments imposed on children with disorders of sex differentiation where they are not vital to the child's health, as noted above.

To the question 'For the purposes of international competition, how ought one to define femaleness or womanhood?' our answer is that it is fair to be considered a woman in competition when one is legally recognised as such. This answer is in line with the recent article that appeared in *JAMA*, authored by Genel, Simpson and de la Chapelle (three clinicians historically involved in IOC and IAAF policies), which supports this view: 'One of the fundamental recommendations published almost 25 years ago that athletes born with a disorder of sex development and raised as females be allowed to compete as women remains appropriate' (Genel et al. 2016).

Moving beyond the cases discussed in this chapter and broadening our analytical gaze, we can see that in elite sport, where discourses of fairness and fair play are reproduced every day, women are still not allowed to participate with the same rules – for example in baseball, soccer, hockey and other sports – where we uphold gender segregation on the basis of some kind of 'different way of playing of women' which is an obviously pejorative historical construction, and a reiteration of gender performativity in sport (Edwards and Jones 2009). Much more work is needed to move this area forward, but for it to be successful, we suspect, sports administrators, ethicists, lawyers and, of course, medical clinicians and researchers will need to work hand in hand rejecting the dominance of any one narrative. Offending the dignity of hyperandrogenic women on the arbitrary grounds of biologically inspired fairness should be rejected. If no more respectful solution can be found we should simply allow them to compete as females, with females.

Notes

All websites accessed October 2017.

1 Parts of Sections 8.3–8.5 in this chapter were previously published in a different version in Camporesi and Maugeri (2016). Permission has been sought and obtained from Routledge for reprinting.
2 www.iaaf.org/news/iaaf-news/iaaf-to-introduce-eligibility-rules-for-femal-1
3 http://medical-dictionary.thefreedictionary.com/hyperandrogenism
4 IAAF Regulations Governing Eligibility of Females with Hyperandrogenism to Compete in Women's Competition (2011): www.iaaf.org/about-iaaf/documents/medical
5 The appendix was taken off the IAAF website after the suspension of the regulations in July 2015. They have been uploaded to the co-author's website at https://silviacamporesiresea rchdotorg.files.wordpress.com/2016/08/iaaf-hyperandrogenism-regulations-appendices.pdf
6 http://assembly.coe.int/nw/xml/XRef/Xref-XML2HTML-EN.asp?fileid=20174&lang=en
7 Paragraph 7.4: 'The athlete shall be responsible for complying with her prescribed medical treatment during the period of Return to Competition Monitoring and shall provide the IAAF Medical Department with satisfactory evidence of such compliance, as it may request' (IAAF Regulations Governing Eligibility of Females with Hyperandrogenism to Compete in Women's Competition – In force as from 1 May 2011).
8 Paragraph 6.6: 'The burden of proof shall be on the athlete to establish, where applicable, that she has an androgen resistance such that she derives no competitive advantage from androgen levels in the normal male range and the standard of proof in such a case shall be by a balance of probabilities. In this the policy is one of strict liability as is the case in anti-doping jurisprudence. It is the athlete who must present themselves for competition and training in a non-doped state.'
9 https://sportsflashes.com/en/others/news/-sports-minister-vijay-goel-supports-dutee-chand-in-her-cas-fight/91462.html
10 Court for Arbitration of Sport Interim Award on Hyperandrogenism Regulations, released 27 July 2015, available at www.tas-cas.org/fileadmin/user_upload/Media_Relea se_3759_FINAL.pdf, paragraph 522.
11 www.theguardian.com/sport/2016/aug/11/caster-semenya-sebastian-coe-iaaf-cas-testos terone-olympics
12 www.theguardian.com/sport/2016/aug/11/caster-semenya-sebastian-coe-iaaf-cas-testos terone-olympics
13 One of the authors, Camporesi, has a manuscript currently under review for the *British Journal of Sport Medicine*, co-authored with Simon Franklin and Jonathan Ospina Betan-curt, that analyses Bermon and Garnier's methodology in terms of robustness and replicability, and interpretation of the data. In re-analysing the results of Bermon and Garnier's paper we applied a correction procedure that controls the false discovery rate, and demonstrate that their results are not robust enough to conclude that they did not arise by chance.

References

All websites accessed October 2017.

Bermon, S. and P.Y. Garnier. 2017. Serum androgen levels and their relation to performance in track and field: mass spectrometry results from 2127 observations in male and female elite athletes. *British Journal of Sports Medicine*, bjsports-2017.

Bermon, S., M. Ritzén, A.L. Hirschberg and T.H. Murray. 2013. Are the new policies on hyperandrogenism in elite female athletes really out of bounds? Response to 'Out of bounds? A critique of the new policies on hyperandrogenism in elite female athletes'. *The American Journal of Bioethics*, 13(5): 63–65.

Bostwick, J.M. and M.J. Joyner. 2012. The limits of acceptable biological variation in elite athletes: should sex ambiguity be treated differently from other advantageous genetic traits? *Mayo Clinic Proceedings*, 87(6): 508–513.

Brunet, L. and M. Salle. 2016. Categorizing and attributing the sex of individuals. In *Gender Testing in Sport: Ethics, Cases and Controversies*, eds S. Montañola and A. Olivesi. New York: Routledge, p. 60–88.

Butler, J. 1990. *Gender Trouble: Feminism and the Subversion of Gender*. New York: Routledge.

Camporesi, S. 2016. Ethics of regulating competition for women with hyperandrogenism. *Clinics in Sports Medicine*, 35(2): 293–301.

Camporesi, S. 2017. Who is a sportswoman? *AEON*, 28 February. Available at: https://aeon.co/essays/sports-culture-binds-us-to-gender-binaries-this-is-unfair

Camporesi, S. and P. Maugeri. 2010. Caster Semenya: sport, categories and the creative role of ethics. *Journal of Medical Ethics*, 36(6): 378–379.

Camporesi, S. and P. Maugeri. 2016. Unfair advantage and the myth of the level playing field in IAAF and IOC policies on hyperandrogenism: when is it fair to be a woman? In *Gender Testing in Sport: Ethics, Cases and Controversies*, eds S. Montañola and A. Olivesi. New York: Routledge, pp. 46–59.

Clarey, C. and G. Kolata. 2009. Gold is awarded amid dispute over runner's sex. *New York Times*, 20 August. Available at: www.nytimes.com/2009/08/21/sports/21runner.html

Cooky, C. and S.L. Dworkin. 2013. Policing the boundaries of sex: a critical examination of gender verification and the Caster Semenya controversy. *Journal of Sex Research*, 50(2): 103–111.

Cooky, C., R. Dycus and S.L. Dworkin. 2013. 'What makes a woman a woman?' versus 'Our first lady of sport': a comparative analysis of the United States and the South African media coverage of Caster Semenya. *Journal of Sport and Social Issues*, 37(1): 31–56.

Daniels, D.B. 1992. Gender (body) verification (building). *Play & Culture*, 5(4): 370–376.

Edwards, K.E. and S.R. Jones. 2009. 'Putting my man face on': a grounded theory of college men's gender identity development. *Journal of College Student Development*, 50(2): 210–228.

Elsas, L.J., A. Ljungqvist, M.A. Ferguson-Smith, J.L. Simpson, M. Genel, A.S. Carlson … and A.A. Ehrhardt. 2000. Gender verification of female athletes. *Genetics in Medicine*, 2(4): 249–254.

Fénichel, P., F. Paris, P. Philibert, S. Hiéronimus, L. Gaspari, J.Y. Kurzenne, P. Chevallier, S. Bermon, N. Chevalier and C. Sultan. 2013. Molecular diagnosis of 5α-reductase deficiency in 4 elite young female athletes through hormonal screening for hyperandrogenism. *The Journal of Clinical Endocrinology & Metabolism*, 98(6): E1055–E1059.

Genel, M., J.L. Simpson and A. de la Chapelle. 2016. The Olympic Games and athletic sex assignment. *JAMA*, 316(13): 1359–1360.

Hämäläinen, M. 2012. The concept of advantage in sport. *Sport, Ethics and Philosophy*, 6(3): 308–322.

Harper, J. 2017. Using testosterone to categorise male and female athletes isn't perfect, but it's the best solution we have. *Guardian*, 3 July. Available at: www.theguardian.com/sport/2017/jul/03/using-testosterone-to-categorise-male-and-female-athletes-isnt-perfect-but-its-the-best-solution-we-have

Hay, E. 1974. Femininity tests at the Olympic Games. *Olympic Review.* 76–77.

Heggie, V. 2010. Testing sex and gender in sports: reinventing, reimagining and reconstructing histories. *Endeavour*, 34(4): 157–163.

Heggie, V. 2011. *A History of British Sports Medicine*. Manchester: Manchester University Press.

Hindustan Times. 2017. Dutee Chand's 'gender case' to be re-opened, IAAF to return to CAS. Available at: www.hindustantimes.com/other-sports/dutee-chand-s-gender-case-to-be-re-opened-iaaf-to-return-to-cas/story-vqQ77jYyIECGaJkIksiVTI.html

Housman, E. and R.V. Reynolds. 2014. Polycystic ovary syndrome: a review for dermatologists: Part I. Diagnosis and manifestations. *Journal of the American Academy of Dermatology*, 71(5): 847–e1.

IAAF. 2015. Press release commenting on CAS suspension of hyperandrogenism regulations. Available at: www.iaaf.org/news/press-release/hyperandrogenism-regulations-cas-dutee-chand

Karkazis, K. and R. Jordan-Young. 2013. The Harrison Bergeron Olympics. *The American Journal of Bioethics*, 13(5): 66–69.

Karkazis, K., R. Jordan-Young, G. Davis and S. Camporesi. 2012. Out of bounds? A critique of the new policies on hyperandrogenism in elite female athletes. *The American Journal of Bioethics*, 12(7): 3–16.

Levy, A. 2009. Either/or. *New Yorker*, 30 November. Available at: www.newyorker.com/magazine/2009/11/30/eitheror

Loland, S. 2002. *Fair Play in Sport: A Moral Norm System*. New York: Routledge.

Loland, S. and H. Hoppeler. 2012. Justifying anti-doping: the fair opportunity principle and the biology of performance enhancement. *European Journal of Sport Science*, 12(4): 347–353.

Lyons, D. 1975. Welcome threats and coercive offers. *Philosophy*, 50(194): 425–436.

Macur, J. 2014. Fighting for the body she was born with. *The New York Times*, 6 October. Available at: www.nytimes.com/2014/10/07/sports/sprinter-dutee-chand-fights-ban-over-her-testosterone-level.html?_r=0

Martínez-Patiño, M.J. 2005. Personal account: a woman tried and tested. *The Lancet*, 366: S38.

Montañola, S. and A. Olivesi, eds. 2016. *Gender Testing in Sport: Ethics, Cases and Controversies*. London: Routledge.

Murray, T.H. 2009. In search of an ethics of sport: genetic hierarchies, handicappers general, and embodied excellence. In *Performance-Enhancing Technologies in Sports*, eds T.H. Murray, K.J. Maschke and A.A. Wasunna. Baltimore, MD: Johns Hopkins University Press, pp. 225–238.

Pielke, R. 2016. *The Edge: The War against Cheating and Corruption in the Cutthroat World of Elite Sports*. Berkeley, CA: Roaring Forties Press.

Pierson, S.T. 2011. The culture of the elite athlete: an enhanced perspective on the case of Caster Semenya, and gender verification testing. *Journal of Genetic Counseling*, 20(3): 323–324.

Rose, F. 2016. Caster Semenya and the intersex hypothesis. In *Gender Testing in Sport: Ethics, Cases and Controversies*, eds S. Montañola and A. Olivesi. New York: Routledge, pp. 101–117.

Schneider, A.J. 2000. On the definition of 'woman' in the sport context. In *Values in Sport: Elitism, Nationalism, Gender Equality and the Scientific Manufacture of Winners*, eds C. Tamburrini and T. Tännsjö. London: Routledge, pp. 123–138.

Schultz, J. 2012. New standards, same refrain: the IAAF's regulations on hyperandrogenism. *The American Journal of Bioethics*, 12(7): 32–33.

Shani, R. and Y.M. Barilan. 2012. Excellence, deviance, and gender: lessons from the XYY episode. *The American Journal of Bioethics*, 12(7): 27–30.

Sherwin, S. and M. Schwartz. 2005. Resisting the emergence of Bio-Amazons. In *Genetic Technology and Sport: Ethical Questions*, eds C. Tamburrini and T. Tännsjö. London: Routledge, p. 199.

Sirmans, S.M. and K.A. Pate. 2014. Epidemiology, diagnosis, and management of polycystic ovary syndrome. *Clinical Epidemiology*, 6(1): 1–13.

Skirstad, B. 2000. Gender verification in competitive sport. In *Values in Sport: Elitism, Nationalism, Gender Equality and the Scientific Manufacture of Winners*, eds C. Tamburrini and T. Tännsjö. London: Routledge, pp. 116–122.

Teetzel, S. 2014. The onus of inclusivity: sport policies and the enforcement of the women's category in sport. *Journal of the Philosophy of Sport*, 41(1): 113–127.

Yang, J.H., L.S. Baskin and M. DiSandro. 2010. Gender identity in disorders of sex development. *Urology*, 75(1): 153–159.

9

CONGENITAL AND ACQUIRED DISABILITIES: WHAT COUNTS AS UNFAIR ADVANTAGE IN THE PARALYMPICS?

9.1 Classification of disability in the Paralympics

The leading body of disability sport, the International Paralympic Committee (IPC), is the counterpart to the IOC in matters of disability sport. It organises a quadrennial event that has grown sufficiently in size and stature that it is no longer considered a mere appendage to the Olympic Games. This may in part be due to the boost to the movement that can be dated back to the Beijing 2008 games, where both events were held in close temporal proximity and utilised the same stadiums and sporting media apparatus. Unlike the IOC, which has had more than a century of global sporting hegemony over all elite able-bodied sports and their respective international federations, the IPC does not comprise all disability sport federations. Specifically, its summer sport programme comprises archery, badminton, boccia, canoe, cycling, equestrian, football five-a-side, goalball, judo, para athletics, para dance sport, para powerlifting, para-swimming, rowing, shooting para-sport, sitting volleyball, table tennis, taekwondo, triathlon, wheelchair basketball, wheel-chair fencing, wheelchair rugby and wheelchair tennis. Six sports comprise the Winter Paralympics: para-alpine skiing, para biathlon, para cross-country skiing, para ice hockey, para-snowboard and wheelchair curling.[1]

In the Paralympics, athletes are grouped by the degree of activity limitation resulting from their impairment(s). The full catalogue of sports, no less than the Paralympic one, celebrates different natural abilities: how embodied capacities (genetically and phenotypically acquired) meet artificial challenges to run, jump and throw, roll and ride, tussle, slide and so on. Each para sport's demands are met by athletes who themselves have functions and activity limitations, which are classified in a sport-specific way.

As asserted by the IPC, the rationale for a sport class, or category, is one of fairness and of ensuring competition. 'A sport class groups athletes with a similar activity limitation together for competition, so that they can compete equitably' (IPC 2017). The original rationale for the organisation in categories of Paralympic sport was to encourage participation in sport by disabled persons, in line with an agenda to integrate people with disabilities into sport (Jones and Howe 2005, 134). A panel of three 'classifiers' (which normally includes a medical doctor and a sport technician) evaluates each athlete. The classifiers work with specific guidelines (a 'functional classification system') that are designed to 'categorise or classify individual sporting participants by their ability to undertake certain physical tasks' (ibid., 137). The physical tasks are general ones that are intended to provide some operational measure of function or ability.

The classification follows the three criteria:

1.   Does the athlete have an eligible impairment for this sport?
2.   Does the athlete's eligible impairment meet the minimum disability criteria of the sport?
3.   Which sport class describes the athlete's activity limitation most accurately?

By 'eligible impairment', it is understood as one of ten impairments identified in the 'Policy on Eligible Impairments in the Paralympic Movement'. The list is found under section 2, chapter 3.13 of the IPC Handbook and is reported in the appendix of this chapter.[2] In addition, each sport's Paralympic classification rules describe how severe an eligible impairment must be, related to the sport context, for an athlete to be considered eligible. These criteria are referred to as 'minimum disability criteria'. Examples of minimum disability criteria could be maximum height for short stature, or degree of amputation of a particular limb. Minor quantitative differences here can literally mean moving from the best in class of one category to the worst in class of another. They are often hotly disputed. Clearly this is a deeply contentious issue which requires enormous trust in the integrity of the evaluation and the evaluator. In order to achieve standardisation, athletes are always assessed before competition and sometimes during competition. Athletes can also be assessed multiple times in their careers, as their impairment may change. This means that athletes may elect to change the category in which they can compete or may be forced to do so. If an athlete meets the criteria for 'minimum disability' for a particular sport, they are eligible to compete in that sport. It may turn out that an athlete may be eligible to compete in one sport, but not in another. Being short can be either a disadvantage or an advantage, depending on the sport: usually it is regarded as an advantage in gymnastics, while in other sports such as basketball being tall is a significant advantage. And, of course, it is no different in life. A relational model of disability calls for an attention not to a deficit, but to the functional limitations resulting from impairments in relation to particular contexts. Thus, classification – which is the central ethical problem of Paralympic sport according to Howe and Jones (2006) – attempts to cater for impairment and sporting contexts in order to generate fair classifications within and between disability groupings. There is only one exception: visual impairment. In the case of visually impaired athletes the classificatory system is a medical system and the sport class allocated therefore applies across all sports (Tweedy and Vanlandewijck 2011).

Note there is currently no rule that prohibits athletes who compete in the Paralympics to compete in the Olympics too. Indeed, there is quite a long list of athletes who have participated in both Olympics and Paralympics, well before South African runner Oscar Pistorius made the headlines in 2008 with his bid to run with able-bodied athletes at the Beijing Olympics. Though unsuccessful then, Pistorius eventually competed with able-bodied athletes at the 2012 London Olympics (see Section 9.4 below). The list of athletes who have been included in both events includes archers, table tennis players, runners, swimmers and equestrians. Examples include[3] the American George Eyser, who won a gold medal in gymnastics while competing on a wooden leg at the 1904 games in St Louis; the New Zealander Neroli Fairhall, paraplegic, who competed in archery in the 1984 Olympics in Los Angeles; Marla Runyan, a legally blind runner from the United States, who competed in the 1500 metres at the 2000 Olympics in Sydney; South African swimmer Natalie du Toit, who in 2008 became the first amputee ever to qualify for the Olympics (Beijing), where she placed 16th in the 10-km 'marathon' swim (Marcellini et al. 2012). In comparison with the recent controversial cases of Pistorius and Rehm discussed below, the participation of many of these athletes in the Olympics has not generated significant debate. As Baker puts it:

> Eyser's accomplishments are highly celebrated, including pop culture references such as a third place ranking in Rolling Stone Magazine's 'Top 100 Greatest Olympians' [...] Likewise, professional archers Neroli Fairhall of New Zealand and Paola Fantato of Italy, each competed in Olympic archery events from a seated position while using a wheelchair and neither faced notable public scrutiny or sanction.
>
> *(Baker 2016, 99–100)*

There are also other uncontroversial examples of athletes identified as disabled who chose not to use available assistive technology (AT) to compete against athletes identified as able-bodied, for example the already mentioned above Natalie du Toit from South Africa (missing left leg) who competed in the 2008 Olympics open water 10 km swim without the use of a prosthetic limb. Another South African, Natalia Partyka, with a right forearm and hand absence, has competed in table tennis in both Olympics and Paralympics. Nevertheless, no Paralympic athlete has ever won a medal at both the Olympic and Paralympic games, although Pistorius earned a silver medal in the 2011 Athletics World Championships by virtue of running a preliminary leg in the South African 4 x 400 m relay team.[4] He was somewhat controversially omitted from the line-up of the relay team.

To what extent is the impaired/able distinction an ontological one? After all, many of us might be considered 'disabled' by virtue of ageing or illness, yet this does not seem to fit with traditional categories. And if the boundaries are permeable, why is that some athletes from disability or Paralympic sports who wish to compete with able-bodied athletes raise controversies in some cases, while not in others? Does the answer lie in the level of performance achieved by the disabled athlete? Baker suggests this might be the case: 'If an individual is not perceived to use his/her AT or disability to get ahead of the game, there is little or no controversy' (Baker 2016, 100). Or might the answer lie in how the AT influences the nature of the activity? Edwards (2008) suggests this might be the case. Before addressing these questions head-on (Section 9.5) it is necessary to do some conceptual groundwork.

9.2 Models of disability and impairment

What is disability? What is impairment? These questions arise because in everyday parlance the concepts are treated as synonyms, and their differences elided. In social and medical philosophy there is a long-standing controversy around the definition of disability, and around the relationships between the two terms. At one extreme are definitions that imply that biological impairments are the sole causes of limitations, while at the other extreme are definitions that attribute the limitations solely to society and characterise disability in terms of exclusion and social oppression. These are often labelled the medical or the social models of disability, but in truth it is an unjustifiable essentialism to represent them as unified schools of thought or paradigms (Jespersen and McNamee 2008). In between are definitions that assert that individual impairment and social environment are jointly sufficient causes of limitation (e.g. WHO International Classification of Functioning, Disability and Health 2001).

According to Jonathan Glover, all disabilities involve some functional limitation (Glover 2006), and this functional limitation distinguishes them from social disadvantage (with the aim to distinguish disability from gender/race or other causes of oppression/exclusion). Naturally, not all philosophers agree. For example, Michael Oliver (the originator of the 'social model of disability': Oliver 1990, 1996, 2013), Gregory Wolbring (2008) and Rosemarie Garland-Thomson (2011, 2014) hold that impairment is social too, and people become disabled only when they encounter a certain context. It was in this vein that Garland-Thomson famously wrote the essay 'The story of my work: how I became disabled' (Garland-Thomson 2014). Whatever the classificatory impulse, impairments are generally seen as traits that the individual cannot readily alter. In general, we could say that what makes a condition an impairment is debatable but it needs to be a stable, long-term condition. The notion of a 'limitation' is also broad and elastic, encompassing restrictions from basic physical activities to more complex social activities. In any case, a limitation must be something that can be measured or assessed. A brief presentation of the different models of disability and impairment is necessary here to understand the rationale for the Paralympic classification:

The medical model of disability was the prevalent model throughout the 1980s and until the early 1990s. An example was the definition put forward by the

World Health Organization (WHO) in 1980, according to which disability is 'any restriction or lack of ability resulting from an impairment to perform an activity in the manner or within the range considered normal for a human being'.[5] The medical model understands a disability as a physical or mental impairment of the individual and the personal and social consequences that go with it, e.g. a defect in the visual system that leads to blindness, a defect in the auditory system that leads to deafness, or a stroke that may lead to speech or movement defects. The medical model regards the limitations faced by people with disabilities as resulting primarily or solely from their impairment, and regards the limitations that result from it as a problem that should be fixed/normalised at the level of the individual (it is against this background of 'ableism' that the advocates of the social model of disability argue). We can see how the medical model is aligned to Boorse's biostatistical theory of health as typical species functioning, discussed in this volume in Chapter 6 as the basis of the therapy/enhancement distinction (Boorse 1977). And we saw the kind of regulatory work it could be put to in anti-doping debates.

In contrast to the medical model, the social model of disability understands disability as a relation between an individual and her social environment. This relation results in the exclusion of people with certain physical and mental characteristics from major domains of life. As put by Oliver (1990), 'Defining impairment or disability or illness is not simply a matter of language, it is a matter of politics and inclusion'. The social model was in the 1990s the bedrock of disability activism, advocating for society to assume responsibility for removing barriers and accepting that impaired persons are not to be considered along the normal/pathological binary, but rather as just one instance of human diversity and of equal value. Disability activists have pushed for the de-medicalisation of disability in many contexts. Its *leitmotif* is that we should change society, not people. Now of course, if one is to change society one must change people and in particular people with disabling attitudes and biases towards those with impairments.

There are more moderate and more extreme versions of the social model of disability. Some of the more extreme activists deny any causal role of impairment to disability but have been heavily criticised, including by disability scholars and activists such as Tom Shakespeare. Shakespeare, who is affected by achondroplasia, or genetic dwarfism, and other related co-morbidities, argues that this is disability in denial: he writes that although disability is often an important/inescapable part of the identity of individuals affected, an approach that denies impairment any causality in the functional limitations is too narrow, and does not capture the complexity of disabled people's lives. That is why, although disability is an 'identity issue', it still remains a health issue, since people with disabilities have greater health needs than the majority of the population. Shakespeare reconceptualises disability, describing persons with disabilities as experiencing a 'narrower margin of health' (Shakespeare 2012, 30). Along the lines of Glover's arguments, he adds that if the disability concept becomes detached from the health component it becomes a generic term of social exclusion (comparable to gender, or race) and loses some of its specific content (Shakespeare 2013).

The bio–psycho–social model recognises that disability cannot be simply equated with impairment, as disability is more than a medically conceived health issue. However, the bio–psycho–social model recognises that impairments are at least partially causative of functional limitations and health needs generally above those of the average population. Also known as the ICF model of disability (WHO International Classification of Functioning, Disability and Health), this model was approved for use by the World Health Assembly in 2001 and defines disability as 'a dynamic interaction between health conditions and environmental and personal factors'. According to the ICF, an impairment is a loss or abnormality of psycho-logical, physiological or anatomical structure or function, while a disability is a restriction or lack (resulting from impairment) of ability to perform an activity in the manner or range that is considered normal for a human being. In so doing, the model integrates different levels in an overall assessment of functional limitations for individuals with disabilities:

1. body functions and structures and impairment thereof;
2. activity of people and activity limitations they experience (such as problems walking up stairs);
3. participation or involvement of people in all areas of life and the participation restriction that they experience (i.e. functioning of a person as a member of society);
4. environmental factors that affect these experiences (facilitators or barriers);
5. personal factors (age, gender, status).

The ICF model has the advantage of being able to offer a guide for the measurement of functional limitations, and is currently the most widely used model for disability. It offers a framework that can be operationalised in clinical practice in many different contexts, from chronic illnesses to rehabilitation medicine, and to the assessment of frailty in older patients (Stucki et al. 2002; Üstün et al. 2003).

Figure 9.1 identifies the three levels of human functioning classified by ICF: functioning at the level of body or body part, the whole person, and the whole person in a social context. Disability therefore involves dysfunctioning at one or more of these same levels: impairments, activity limitations and participation restrictions.

Among the contextual factors that can be listed are external environmental factors (such as social attitudes, characteristics of the built environment, legal and social structures, as well as climate, terrain and so forth); and subjective factors, which include gender, age, coping styles, social background, education, profession, past and current experience, overall behaviour pattern, character and other factors that influence how disability is experienced by the individual. Reverberations of the bio–psycho–social model can also be found in the 2001 Convention on the Rights of Persons with Disabilities (UN 2001), which defines disability as 'an evolving concept' that 'results from the interaction between persons with impairments and attitudinal and environmental barriers that hinders their full and effective

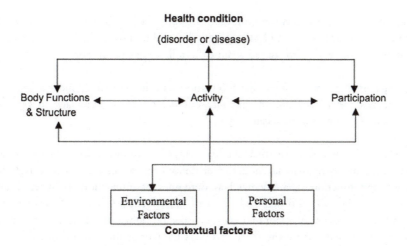

FIGURE 9.1 The three levels of human functioning classified by the ICF
(Adapted from www.who.int/classifications/icf/icfbeginnersguide.pdf?ua=1)

participation in society on an equal basis with others'. This conception can also be found at work in the IPC classification, as outlined in the next section.

The medical community has arguably been slower in moving beyond the model of disability from which its name arises. Important strides have been made in this direction in the last ten years, especially since the 2009 *Lancet* special issue entirely dedicated to disability, which defined people with disabilities as 'individuals who do not all think and act according to the "disabled" label that society has assigned them' (*The Lancet* 2009, 1793) and urges health professionals and policy-makers to 'take note' (ibid.). Another noteworthy feature of the 2009 *Lancet* special issue was its explicit alignment with the International Classification of Functioning, Disability and Health and with the UN Convention on the Rights of Persons with Disabilities (adopted 2006) to view disability as the outcome of complex interactions between health conditions and the physical and social environment, and urging for revised training of health professionals in this light (Shakespeare et al. 2009; Stein et al. 2009).

9.3 Theoretical underpinnings of Paralympics classification

As stated by the IPC, classes or categories exist in the Paralympics for two reasons: (a) to ensure inclusiveness allowing the participation of individuals with relevant impairments; (b) to ensure fairness of opportunity and some kind of level playing field so that athletes within the same category can compete equitably. Thus the IPC writes: 'A sport class groups athletes with a similar activity limitation together for competition, so that they can compete equitably' (IPC 2017). As noted in Section 9.1, there are three necessary steps to classify an athlete as eligible to compete in a particular Paralympic category, i.e. whether an athlete has an eligible impairment for the particular sport for which she is being assessed; whether the eligible impairment meets the minimum disability criteria for the sport; and which sport class describes the athlete's activity limitation most accurately. Hence, an athlete's impairment is measured against the following two criteria:

a against a specific context (sport demands, with its rules etc.); and
b against specific minimum disability criteria, which are in place to preserve competitiveness in that category.

We could therefore say that the Paralympic Committee adopts to a certain extent the bio-psycho-social model of disability of impairment, in which ICF disability and functioning are viewed as outcomes of interactions between health conditions (diseases, disorders and injuries) and contextual factors. Moreover, the contextual factors vary according to sport-specific demands. Hence, in the measurements carried out by the three classifiers limitations they are measured against the minimum disability criteria to ensure competitiveness within a certain category.

Among the contextual factors we can also count whether the disability is congenital or acquired, as that may generate a difference for the resulting performance. We have noted that there are broadly speaking two categories of athletes competing in the Paralympics:

a Athletes with a congenital disability, i.e. present from birth; and
b Athletes with an acquired disability for which an equivalent (phenotypically) disability exists, but with a different etiological (congenital) basis.

Note that while often a congenital condition would have a genetic basis, there can be instances of congenital conditions that are caused by the maternal or external environment (e.g. fetal alcohol syndrome), although of course to some extent all disabilities have a genetic basis (some noxious stimulus in the environment would trigger some genetic/epigenetic pathway leading to the phenotypic manifestation of the disability). American athlete Maria Runyan is an example of the former category: she was diagnosed with progressive vision loss as a child, and her condition was present since birth. Italian archer Paola Fantato is an example of the latter: she contracted poliomyelitis when she was a child and ended up in a wheelchair: she competed at the Atlanta Olympics in 1996. Maria Runyan was the first legally blind athlete able to qualify for the US Olympic Team in 2000 in the 1500 metres event. She went on to compete in the 2000 and 2004 Olympics.

There is anecdotal evidence that athletes with congenital disabilities are typically outperformed by athletes with acquired disabilities. Moreover, there is anecdotal evidence that many countries seek out athletes with newly acquired impairments in the hope of greater performance results.[6] The reasons are not entirely clear, and there is no systematic research basis for the judgement, though it is widely believed that those who have already developed through skill and other capacity development in life, having acquired a disability later in life, have a distinct competitive advantage. While data are available in basketball (Skordilis et al. 2006), and are consistent with achievements of individuals with congenital disabilities in other contexts different from sport, there are no data to the best of our knowledge in other sports. Extrapolating from these data and from the evidence that countries seek out athletes with newly acquired impairments in the hope of better performance results, a case could be made that Runyan progressively adjusted herself to her disabilities, having been diagnosed when she was 10 years old. Thus it might be inferred that she had the advantage of having started to run, and develop the relevant motoric skills, when she was still sighted. To the best of our knowledge there are no examples of athletes who are congenitally blind that ran (or indeed could run) in the Olympics at the required level given minimum performance eligibility requirements.

One question which is open for discussion and that we briefly touch upon below is whether these athletes ought to compete directly against each other within the same class. We note that the second criterion of the IPC is that of fair opportunity – what they call 'competitiveness'. But ought the IPC to generate two classes on the basis of the different etiology of the same condition?

At present this is not considered to be a relevant distinction by the IPC. Peter van der Vliet, the IPC's medical and science director, puts it thus:

> I am not aware of any examples in any sport where congenital deficits (dysmelia, or limb deficiency) are dealt with separately to traumatic amputation, by nature of the concept of classification. This is: we assess the impact of an impairment on activity, rather than the origin of an impairment as a classification criteria. But I would agree with you that one needs to be sensitive towards, and preferably avoid, recruitment of newly acquired impairment athletes. On the one hand there is an increased number of such cases (e.g. preventive amputation of lower limbs for bone cancer, traumatic accidents with higher survival ratios, increased post trauma care and rehabilitation) as well as due to 'easy access' recruitment bases (e.g. rehabilitation hospitals) and (a moral obligation to) invest in post-trauma care (e.g. war veteran activity programs). Anecdotal evidence also indicates a preference from certain coaches towards war veterans because of their attitude towards (training) regimen and their group/team spirit. We not only see this in war veterans, but also in the coordination impairment categories where there is an increasing number of traumatic brain injury athletes over the historical CP (cerebral palsy) population.
>
> *(Van de Vliet, personal correspondence, 20 July 2017)*

What, if anything, could we do to redress this discrepancy in performance between athletes with congenital and acquired disabilities? There could be two routes: one might be to construct more categories and divide athletes on the basis of the cause of their condition (this is the 'distinguishing populations on grounds of fairness' strategy). The latter would be to augment the genetic impairment with technology to redress the unfairness. This latter strategy might be analogous to Tamburrini and Tännsjö's attempts to argue for the genetic engineering of athlete 'bio-Amazons' to facilitate equality of opportunity as a case in point (Tamburrini and Tännsjö 2005). Jones and Howe (2005) suggest that disability sports should adopt the dominant view in philosophy of sport i.e. that both the constitutive rules of a certain sport and the prevailing ethos should provide competitors the 'level playing field', and ensure that the victory goes to whoever 'merits' it most (Loland and McNamee 2000). From this it would follow that rules should therefore limit the effects of chance and remove as much as possible the obstacles that 'preclude the realization of fair and meritocratic victories' (Jones and Howe 2005, 136). Jones and Howe also point out some inherent limitations in the IPC functional classification system, the major problem being that it does not consider 'training effects' on a competitor's ability. Specifically they point to the difficulty in arbitrating with any degree of precision the extent to which we can practically disentangle 'aspects of athletic performance for which one cannot claim responsibility' (i.e. an unmerited baseline physical capacity) from aspects of athletic performance for which one may claim responsibility/merit (e.g. resulting from training). We note how this is not just a practical difficulty, as it mirrors an underlying conceptual problem when trying to 'cleave athletic performance along chance and merit line' (ibid., 142).

To sum up, the philosophical challenge for the IPC functional classification system seems to be striking a balance between creating enough classes that it can achieve some sort of level playing field within each class, without having so many that they are reduced to 'idiosyncratic comparisons of minute differences in physical function' (ibid., 142). And of course, there is a more prosaic one, i.e. just how many classes can one have in an event given the pressures of scheduling and the need for (time-consuming) medal ceremonies. Though not a philosophical point, it is an undeniably important one: it raises matters of media-driven commercialisation where the Paralympic sport development model has been based on the successes of the Olympic sponsor- and mediatised-driven model. We leave that one, however, for our more sociologically informed colleagues.

In the next section we compare two cases of Paralympic athletes who have recently challenged international bodies to compete with able-bodied athletes, the former with a congenital, the latter with an acquired disability. It is important to discuss these cases to explicate the theoretical underpinning regarding the debate about unfair advantage in the Paralympics.

9.4 Congenital versus acquired disabilities: Pistorius versus Rehm

A recent famous, turned infamous, example of an athlete with a congenital disability bidding to compete in the Olympics is the case of Oscar Pistorius (Camporesi 2008; Burkett et al. 2011; Marcellini et al. 2012). Oscar Pistorius was born on 22 November 1986 without fibulae (the outer bones between the knee and the ankle) due to a genetic condition, and had both legs amputated below the knee when he was 11 months old. Pistorius was reported saying: 'I grew up not really thinking I had a disability, I grew up thinking I had different shoes' (Moreton 2012).

Pistorius used to run with the aid of carbon-fibre artificial limbs produced by the Icelandic company Össur, called 'Cheetahs'. In 2007 Pistorius took part in his first international competition for able-bodied athletes, first in his home country of

South Africa, then in Rome, Italy. At that time, the IAAF temporarily allowed him to compete with able-bodied athletes, while performing tests on the prosthesis. The IAAF assigned to German Professor Gert-Peter Brüggemann (director of the Institute of Biomechanics and Orthopaedics, German Sport University Cologne) the task of monitoring Oscar's performances and analysing the information, which the IAAF would then use as the empirical basis for its decision. Brüggemann's study concluded that Pistorius's limbs used 25 per cent less energy than able-bodied athletes to run at the same speed and the prosthetic limbs developed an energy loss of about 9% during the stance phase, compared with 41% in the human ankle joint (Brüggemann et al. 2008). Based on these findings, Brüggemann concluded that Pistorius was actually performing a 'different kind of locomotion at lower metabolic cost' (ibid., 227). On the strength of these findings, on 14 January 2008, the IAAF ruled Pistorius ineligible for competitions conducted under its rules, including the 2008 Beijing Summer Olympics. In the same year, the IAAF amended its competition rules to ban the use of 'any technical device that incorporates springs, wheels or any other element that provides a user with an advantage over another athlete not using such a device' (rule 144.2). The federation claimed that the amendment was not specifically aimed at Pistorius.

Following the IAAF decision, Pistorius appealed to the Court of Arbitration for Sport (CAS) in Lausanne (since 1984, the place where international sports disputes are resolved). He travelled to the US to take part in a series of further tests carried out at Rice University in Houston, Texas by a team of scientists including Hugh Herr and Rodger Kram. In their point-by-point reply to the work by Brüggemann et al. (2008), Kram et al. (2010) argued that as there were no sufficient data to support the claim that Pistorius had an advantage, the conclusion should be that he does not have an advantage over able-bodied athletes. They wrote: 'Until recently it would have been preposterous to consider prosthetic limbs to be advantageous, thus, the burden of proof is on those who claim that running specific prostheses (RSP) are advantageous' (Kram et al. 2010, 1012).

On the basis of these findings, on 26 May 2008, the CAS in Lausanne reversed the IAAF decision and ruled that Pistorius should be able to compete against Olympic athletes, since the IAAF 'did not prove that claim [of unfair advantage] to a sufficient extent' (Arbitration CAS 2008/A/1480). Note that the verdict was limited only to the use of the specific blades in issue in this appeal (that is, were Pistorius to change the kind of running-specific prosthesis he used, he would have to go through the same testing regimen again). It was therefore a very contextualised decision that could not be extended to other double amputees, who – according to the IAAF – would also have to undertake the relevant biomechanical tests. After the appeal to CAS, Pistorius was allowed to compete with able-bodied athletes. Although he was not able to qualify for the Beijing games in the summer of 2008, he was the first amputee to compete in track events at the Olympics Games in London 2012, where he advanced to the semi-finals with a time of 46.54 seconds.

Pistorius competed also in the Paralympics in London in 2012. As noted above, his participation in the Olympics did not exclude him from participation in the

Paralympics. As it will be evident from the list of athletes reported at the beginning of this chapter, Oscar Pistorius is not by any means the first case of an athlete with an impairment or 'disability' competing in the Olympics, though he was the first amputee to compete in track events at the Games.

The second example that we would like to discuss in this section is the case of the German Paralympic athlete Markus Rehm. Rehm is a single amputee long-jumper, his disability the result of a boating accident when he was 14 years old (Bloom 2015). Contrary to Pistorius, he has an acquired disability. Rehm made the news when he jumped 8.40 metres at the IPC Championships in Doha in 2015. That jump could have earned him a medal at the London Olympics in 2012. Indeed, it would have beaten the British athlete Greg Rutherford, who won the gold in London with 8.31 metres. Rehm's closest competitor in Doha jumped 6.69 metres (ibid.). Rehm originally declared his intention to compete in the Rio Olympic Games of 2016, but his claims were rejected by the IAAF after 'failing to prove he did not have an unfair advantage'. As with hyperandrogenic athletes discussed in the previous chapter, the IAAF placed the onus on the athlete – in this case to prove that his prosthesis gave him no unfair advantage.[7] However, as we among other philosophers and ethicists of sport have noted, empirical conclusions regarding eligibility are never purely '*technical*' judgements; questions of norms and values contribute to the creation of the evidentiary threshold that constitutes an assessment of evidence or a category (Baker 2016; Camporesi 2008; Marcellini et al. 2012; Camporesi 2015).

A comparative analysis of the two cases sheds light on similarities and differences. Regarding the similarities, we note how (i) there cannot be counterfactual scenarios in either case, i.e. we cannot compare Pistorius running on prostheses with an able-bodied Pistorius, and the same goes for Rehm. This means that to demonstrate that there is no unfair advantage, as required by IAAF, we are left to compare the two athletes against some existing able-bodied norm (see below for a discussion); (ii) both athletes are running on prosthesis/prostheses, which are essential for performance but are also considered performance enhancing and are contested because they are thought to provide an unfair advantage in competition; (iii) both athletes are competing at a level that is much higher than the level of their fellow athletes in the Paralympics. That is why they are bidding to be competing with able-bodied athletes in the Olympics, as that would provide them with that competitive element which is lacking in their own category in the Paralympics. As noted at the beginning of this chapter and also in the previous chapter, categories in sport are constructed to ensure a level playing field and to ensure that competition is retained within such categories.

The differences between Pistorius's and Rehm's cases are the following: (i) most obviously Rehm runs and jumps with one prosthesis, whereas Pistorius uses two prostheses (an atypical case where a greater level of impairment leads *ceteris paribus* to a performance enhancement in stability and efficiency). Is this difference relevant? Well, one could say that it is relevant since Markus Rehm has developed in personal bests very significantly since he began jumping (springing off) from his prosthesis (Beckman et al. 2016). His personal best from his non-prosthetic limb is nearly 90 centimeters less (see below for a more in-depth discussion), which would almost certainly render him ineligible to compete because of inadequate performance in the elite class; (ii) the mode of competition: running (Pistorius) versus long-jumping (Rehm). These are different kinds of activities, which have prompted some scholars to argue that prosthesis changes the nature of the activity of running (Edwards 2008). Although this is the entire event for Pistorius, it is an essential component in the long jump, since speed is converted to height and therefore distance; (iii) Regarding levels of performance: the best result for Pistorius in the 400 metres at the London 2012 Olympics (46.54 seconds) earned him a place in the semi-finals, but Pistorius had never a chance to win an Olympic medal (the current Olympics record is held by another South African, Wayde van Niekerk, with 43.03), which would place compatriot van Niekerk nearly 30 metres ahead of Pistorius if a hypothetical race based on personal bests were imagined. By contrast, Markus Rehm with his 8.40 metres jump in Doha made it very clear that he could have aimed at an Olympic medal.

This difference in levels of performance is relevant, as the IAAF is asking athletes to prove that they have no unfair advantage compared to able-bodied athletes; but because we obviously cannot compare Pistorius and Rehm with their able-bodied selves, we are left to compare them with other able-bodied athletes. If no reference point can be found in an existing able-bodied athlete who runs faster/jumps longer than Pistorius/Rehm, disabled athletes will not be in a position to demonstrate that their prosthesis do not provide them with an unfair advantage.

This, in other words, is the crux of the matter. The question that the IAAF is requiring disabled athletes to answer is the following: does the prosthesis offer them an advantage in competition? What we know is that Rehm's personal best developed very significantly in major athletics events in 2012–2014, increasing by 0.89m as follows:

London, UK 2012: 7.35 m;
Ulm, Germany 2014: 8.24 m;
Doha, Qatar 2015: 8.40 m.

We know that this is a dramatic improvement for one mature in their career, where leaps in performance are often the source of suspicion for reasons of doping. We cannot be clear it was not both the efficiency of the prosthetic and new technical adaptations. We need to question, however, whether that is the right kind of question to ask.

Biomechanical tests have demonstrated that Rehm's jump strategy is based on 'energy storage and return' in prosthetic jumping, while it is based on 'redirecting the movement direction' in jumping with biological legs. We could therefore say – following Edwards (2008) – that jumping off his prosthesis changes to some extent the nature of the activity. Is this a change relevant enough to justify classifying him in a different category? Biomechanical tests have also demonstrated that Rehm has a much more efficient take-off compared to an able-bodied norm, due to use of the prosthesis to spring off (56% vs 113%), although in the run–up the use of the prosthesis might inhibit force and power generation, which might be disadvantageous (*Wolfgang Potthast, personal communication, 29 June 2017*).

It seems to us that these two cases discussed above, among others, prompt a more general ethical consideration of the role of AT in Paralympic sports. Baker (2016) distinguishes three objections:

1. AT being used perceived to afford an unfair advantage (the case of Pistorius and Rehm);
2. AT perceived to threaten the purity of sport; and
3. AT perceived as a precursor to a slippery slope to a morally reprehensible end (such as enhancement, doping).

The assumption underlying the first objections to the use of AT in sport is that quantifiable standards of 'normal' human performance exist. A consequence of this assumption is a 'disproportionate' restriction of individuals with disabilities from the same opportunities to 'achieve greatness as individuals without disabilities' (Baker 2016, 95). That is why, even if it were impossible to prove with biomechanical and/or physiological studies that a disabled athlete does not have an advantage over an able-bodied athlete in the absence of an agreed-upon scientific reference point (as in the case of Markus Rehm), these studies would have difficulty establishing the degree of (potential) enhancement. And precise data are necessary for the ethical evaluation regarding any unfair advantage. Science alone cannot answer the question of what counts as an unfair advantage in competition. Biomechanical and other scientific data are necessary but not sufficient; what counts as a level playing field is not reducible to performance data.

Moreover, we cannot evaluate except against some standard. Here the normal body is taken as a standard, but this opens up the potential charge of ability-bias or 'ableism', as it has been called (Wolbring 2012). The question then becomes: what is this 'standard measure' against which Paralympic performance is being compared? Or, put in other words: how is the 'normal standard' (the norm) measured in competitive sport? However measured, this 'normal standard' is not fixed but evolves over time: when new training regimes or the latest scientific studies allow new records to be broken, then a new piece of equipment (technology) is introduced, and so on and so forth (Fouché 2017).

As Baker points out (2016), it is only when the use of AT is perceived as being potentially performance enhancing that the controversy regarding the eligibility of disabled athletes to compete with able-bodied athletes appears to arise. Certainly, as we noted at the beginning of this chapter, there is a long list of athletes who have competed in both Olympics and Paralympics without sparking any controversy; on the contrary, they were celebrated for their participation. Karpin and Mykitiuk were the first to point out that disabled bodies may not only constitute one 'end' of the Gaussian curve respective to the standard body, but both ends: 'those identified as disabled might simultaneously occupy both ends of the curve at once'

(Karpin and Mykitiuk 2008, 428). They discuss this in the case of an amputee, Aimee Mullins, who is both disabled and a fashion super-model, an amputee and a champion sprinter. To a reasonable degree the same argument is valid also for Oscar Pistorius or Markus Rehm. The important point to make here is that, contrary to public expectations perhaps, able-bodied athletes are not bound to a fixed ceiling of performance, as the 'normal standard' is evolving, while disabled athletes are bound to the 'normal standard' established by able-bodied athletes. Clearly, there is work here for philosophers and scientists to attempt to systematise these judgements, combining the challenging data and argument from biomechanics, physiology and philosophy.

As noted by Baker (2016), even in the case of Oscar Pistorius, although he was ultimately allowed to compete with able-bodied athletes, the CAS decision reinforced the issue of holding him accountable to a 'normal human' standard, by arguing that there was no evidence to prove that he did not have an advantage:

> What is critical here is that, although the stated requirement is that Pistorius 'be permitted to compete on the same footing as others,' the counsel interprets this requirement to mean he will only be allowed to compete if he is found to perform at or below some set of performance standards based on a group of his peers, which is not a restriction that 'able-bodied' athletes are held accountable to [...] Essentially the CAS report allowed Pistorius to compete because they could not prove that his prosthetic legs afforded an unfair advantage, but the emphasis on comparing and restricting Pistorius (and presumably other athletes in a similar situation) to remain at or below a normal standard of performance was reinforced.
>
> *(Baker 2016, 97)*

The question of legality versus legitimacy is a thorny one indeed. Establishing proper norms for comparison is quite exceptionally challenging. We can say that it is unacceptable simple to posit scientific data without recognising some large assumptions about normality. It is plausible to speculate that the CAS will not allow Rehm to compete exactly because of his higher levels of performance/achievements compared to able-bodied athletes. Although a CAS decision will not say so explicitly, it will implicitly contain a value-judgement about what is the normal human body that can provide the adequate reference point. But it must be recognised that such judgements are essentially both multidisciplinary and normative. As with the hyperandrogenism case discussed in the previous chapter, one wonders why adjudicating panels at WADA and the IPC are not comprised of a greater range of expertise including philosophy.

9.5 The value of technology in Paralympic sport

Beckman et al. argue that cases like Pistorius or Rehm raise broader kind of issues such as: 'Ought we to encourage direct competition between people who do and do not require enabling technology in elite-level sports event such as the Olympics?' (Beckman et al. 2016, 1) They also argue, along the lines of what we noted above, that the answer to this question cannot require only a scientific assessment of a technological advantage but needs to include an assessment of philosophical considerations, such as for example: (i) the type of activity the athletes are performing; (ii) whether such differences in activity warrant putting them in a different category; and (iii) whether considerations of 'equity and human dignity' are raised by notions of inclusiveness for people who require enabling technology in the Olympics.

Edwards (2008), as noted above, raises a similar point to the second one in relation to Oscar Pistorius, regarding whether his was not running but high velocity bounding. In other words, he suggests that prosthetics alter the very nature of the activity. Put starkly: are the inevitable biomechanical differences so significant that people who use technology ought to be thought of as performing a different activity from their competitors? In this sense, he argues, the role of technology could be seen as a demarcation line between two types of events, one in which technology plays a prominent role, and one in which it does not.

Tännsjö (2009) offers an equally provocative thought experiment of a high jumper who had genetically engineered legs that were 3 meters tall. Why would we admire his world-record-breaking performances that would merely require him to walk over the bar – requiring little by way of complex technique, effort, training or natural talent? Equally, one would not allow a person with a pole to compete in the high jump competition, but a separate event could be perfectly acceptable, as all athletes would perform under the same parameters and the level playing field would be retained. The question for Oscar Pistorius then becomes: is his movement sufficiently different from running (provided that running is a vague concept or category) to warrant putting him in another category? And in Markus Rehm's case, what constitutes long-jumping, or high-springing? What is that activity that we call long jump and what are the features of excellence of the activity that a blade may impair, or change? And how can we establish that? Along these lines, one could compare bionic and wheelchair racing with the pole vault and other sports where athletes use external tools to move beyond species-typical functioning, while comparing biological racing with the high jump where no such external tools are used. Since both the high jump and the pole vault are included in international athletic events, one might also envisage having both 'high-velocity bounding' and biological running therein, though in a separate class from traditional track events. In other words, going 'beyond species-typical functioning' need not be a reason to exclude amputee athletes from competing in the international able-bodied sports, unless the *raison d'être* or internal values of the events ruled them out by way of conceptual analysis or ethical argument. A discussion of the nature of the activity itself would necessarily include a discussion of the types of excellences intrinsic in a certain practice (something developed by John William Devine in his account of the continued justification of the anti-doping ban – see Devine 2010), and a discussion of the role and value of technology in Paralympic sport.

Burkett, a biomechanist and former Paralympic swimming world champion himself, has written extensively on the value of technology in sports. He argues that technology is in many cases 'essential for performance' in Paralympic sports (Burkett et al. 2011). For example, there are specialised prostheses for athletes who compete in track and field throwing events such as shot-put, javelin and discus, or in jumping events. Similarly, there are specialised wheelchairs to enable athletes to compete in the equivalent of rugby, tennis and basketball. All these technologies, while being essential for performance, are also designed to enhance performance. The two features seem to be inextricably intertwined. The same happens also with the bikes for elite cycling, which are also designed to enhance performance. The point with performance-enhancing technologies in sport seems to be a problem of standardisation of the 'essential for performance-enhancing performance' technology; that is, there needs to be an upper limit or cut-off point (arbitrarily chosen among a series of possible upper limits) for the biotechnology, above which we decide that the value of athletic performance, and our admiration for it, are severely impaired by the technology itself (Murray et al. 2009).

As noted at the beginning of this chapter, two main considerations enter into the International Paralympic Classification: considerations of inclusivity, and considerations of fairness or ensuring a level playing field. In relation to this second point, it seems that the requirement set by the IAAF to put the onus of proof on the disabled athlete to demonstrate that they do not have an unfair advantage is running against inclusivity considerations. A similar point was raised by Teetzel (2014) with respect to hyperandrogenic athletes, as noted in the previous chapter. This is an especially important point considering the financial burden that goes with it. An article that appeared in the German newspaper *Die Zeit* in 2016 entitled 'Markus Rehm: is he better, because he is disabled?' (echoing the title of another article that appeared in the *New York Times* nine years previously titled 'An amputee sprinter: is he disabled, or too abled?' (Longman 2007)), reported that Rehm did not have the financial means to appeal to the CAS or to commission alternative biomechanics studies, contrary to what Pistorius did (Henk 2016), and included an extended interview with Rehm.[8]

Returning to the question, 'which one of the two conceptualisations ("essential for performance" vs "performance enhancing") should prevail in our assessment of the role of biotechnology on our athletic performance', Burkett (2010) argues – rightly in our opinion – that, given that a 'grey area' remains regarding how well an athlete is able to transfer any potential mechanical advantage into a real advantage, we should err on the side of the benefit of the doubt – of inclusivity. Now of course, there are grey areas and there are grey areas, and we would have to estimate responsibly just how ambiguous were the cases in hand and how they challenged existing wisdom (and sporting categories). This implies that we should probably favour technology that is essential for performance, rather than which was merely performance enhancing (Burkett et al.

2011). In this sense, Pistorius is an example of a technological hybrid or a 'compound athlete' (Marcellini et al. 2012) as opposed to some science-fiction cyborg. Clearly, the prosthetic technology enables his performance but also becomes an extension of his embodiment; a point often made – for example – in relation to the greatest of tennis players regarding their rackets. The main problem for evaluating the role of technology, for Burkett, remains the problem of equity of access as highlighted above.

9.6 Conclusions

Questions pertaining to the inclusion of Paralympic athletes in able-bodied categories are complex questions that cannot be settled merely with biomechanical tests. They require a normative discussion of fairness, and of the value of technology in sport, and of the ways, if any, in which assisted technology is changing the nature of the activity itself. Although most congenital abnormalities are genetic, including the case of Oscar Pistorius, there are some congenital abnormalities that are acquired due to external environmental influences during the gestation time. That does not mean they do not have a genetic etiology, as an environmental stimulus necessarily triggers some genetic/epigenetic pathway which leads to the manifestations of a particular condition, disability or syndrome. In this chapter we have not explicitly discussed examples of athletes with a genetic condition/disability who are aspiring to compete in the Olympics for the simple reason that at the moment there are none. We can expect, however that there will be more cases of athletes with congenital abnormalities who will aspire to compete with able-bodied athletes. A serious engagement with the above questions will be necessary to avoid falling prey to a simple reduction of complex questions to scientific or biomechanical answers.

Appendix

List of 10 eligible impairments according to International Paralympic Classification:[9]

1. Impaired muscle power: Reduced force generated by muscles or muscle groups, such as muscles of one limb or the lower half of the body, as caused, for example, by spinal cord injuries, spina bifida or polio.
2. Impaired passive range of movement: Range of movement in one or more joints is reduced permanently, for example due to arthrogryposis. Hypermobility of joints, joint instability and acute conditions, such as arthritis, are not considered eligible impairments.
3. Limb deficiency: Total or partial absence of bones or joints as a consequence of trauma (e.g. car accident), illness (e.g. bone cancer) or congenital limb deficiency (e.g. dysmelia).
4. Leg length difference: Bone shortening in one leg due to congenital deficiency or trauma.

5.   Short stature: Reduced standing height due to abnormal dimensions of bones of upper and lower limbs or trunk, for example due to achondroplasia or growth hormone dysfunction.

6.   Hypertonia: Abnormal increase in muscle tension and a reduced ability of a muscle to stretch, due to a neurological condition, such as cerebral palsy, brain injury or multiple sclerosis.

7.   Ataxia: Lack of coordination of muscle movements due to a neurological condition, such as cerebral palsy, brain injury or multiple sclerosis.

8.   Athetosis: Generally characterised by unbalanced, involuntary movements and a difficulty in maintaining a symmetrical posture, due to a neurological condition, such as cerebral palsy, brain injury or multiple sclerosis.

9.   Visual impairment: Vision is impacted by either an impairment of the eye structure, optical nerves or optical pathways, or the visual cortex.

10.   Intellectual impairment: A limitation in intellectual functioning and adaptive behaviour as expressed in conceptual, social and practical adaptive skills, which originates before 18 years old.

Notes

All websites accessed October 2017.

1   www.paralympic.org/sports
2   www.paralympic.org/sites/default/files/document/130214165045592_IPC+Policy+on+Eligible+Impairments+in+the+Paralympic+Movement.pdf
3   An updated list of athletes who have competed in both Olympics and Paralympic events can be found here: https://en.wikipedia.org/wiki/List_of_athletes_who_have_competed_in_the_Paralympics_and_Olympics
4   www.espn.com/olympics/summer/2012/trackandfield/story/_/id/8250476/2012-london-olympics-oscar-pistorius-4x400-meter-relay-reaches-final-appeal
5   http://apps.who.int/iris/bitstream/10665/41003/1/9241541261_eng.pdf
6   At proofs stage, we became aware of an article by Paul Grant published for BBC Sport on 17 September 2017 that details how Peter Van de Vliet, the IPC's medical and scientific director, reportedly has 'no control' over countries recruiting athletes at the higher end of each disability class, and admitted that 'nations tend to recruit athletes in view of medal chances and financial support that may come from medals at major events and Paralympic Games': www.bbc.co.uk/sport/disability-sport/41253174
7   www.bbc.com/sport/olympics/36565093
8   There is a point to be made here (similar to the one we made in Chapter 8) that the onus of proof that the IAAF puts on athletes to demonstrate absence of advantage is unfair. Markus Rehm does not make a living with earnings from professional sport. During the day he works at a medical centre in Troisdorf near Cologne, as a master of orthopaedic technology. He simply did not have the means to commission expensive biomechanical tests in order to appeal to the CAS to compete in Rio. He seems to have secured a Japanese sponsor (as of April 2016) so he might have the funds to commission biomechanical studies and appeal to the CAS in the future, but did not have thus far (contrary to Pistorius, who was generously sponsored). See www.koelnsport.de/markus-rehm-eine-frage-der-fairness/
9   Reproduced from www.paralympic.org/sites/default/files/document/130214165045592_IPC+Policy+on+Eligible+Impairments+in+the+Paralympic+Movement.pdf

References

All websites accessed October 2017.

Arbitration CAS 2008/A/1480 Pistorius v/ IAAF, award of 16 May 2008. Available at: https://jurisprudence.tas-cas.org/Shared%20Documents/1480.pdf

Baker, D.A. 2016. The 'second place' problem: assistive technology in sports and (re) constructing normal. *Science and Engineering Ethics*, 22(1): 93–110.

Beckman, E.M., M.J. Connick, M.J. McNamee, R. Parnell and S.M. Tweedy. 2016. Should Markus Rehm be permitted to compete in the long jump at the Olympic Games? *British Journal of Sport Medicine*, 51: 1048–1049.

Bloom, B. 2015. Markus Rehm leaps into Rio controversy. *Daily Telegraph*, 23 October. Available at: www.telegraph.co.uk/sport/olympics/paralympic-sport/11952281/IPC-Athletics-World-Championships-Markus-Rehm-leaps-into-Rio-controversy.html

Boorse, C. 1977. Health as a theoretical concept. *Philosophy of Science*, 44(4): 542–573.

Brüggemann, G.P., A. Arampatzis, F. Emrich and W. Potthast. 2008. Biomechanics of double transtibial amputee sprinting using dedicated sprinting prostheses. *Sports Technology*, 1(4–5): 220–227.

Burkett, B. 2010. Technology in Paralympic sport: performance enhancement or essential for performance? *British Journal of Sports Medicine*, 44(3): 215–220.

Burkett, B., M. McNamee and W. Potthast. 2011. Shifting boundaries in sports technology and disability: equal rights or unfair advantage in the case of Oscar Pistorius? *Disability & Society*, 26(5): 643–654.

Camporesi, S. 2008. Oscar Pistorius, enhancement and post-humans. *Journal of Medical Ethics*, 34(9): 639.

Camporesi, S. 2015. Bioethics and sport. In *Routledge Handbook of the Philosophy of Sport*, eds M.J. McNamee and W.J. Morgan. Abingdon: Routledge, pp. 81–97.

Devine, J.W. 2010. Doping is a threat to sporting excellence. *British Journal of Sports Medicine*, 45: 637–639.

Edwards, S.D. 2008. Should Oscar Pistorius be excluded from the 2008 Olympic games? *Sports Ethics and Philosophy*, 2(2): 112–125.

Fouché, R. 2017. *Game Changer: The Technoscientific Revolution in Sports.* Baltimore, MD: Johns Hopkins University Press.

Garland-Thomson, R. 2011. Misfits: a feminist materialist disability concept. *Hypatia*, 26(3): 591–609.

Garland-Thomson, R. 2014. The story of my work: how I became disabled. *Disability Studies Quarterly*, 34(2).

Glover, J. 2006. *Choosing Children: Genes, Disability, and Design.* Oxford: Oxford University Press.

Henk, M. 2016. Is er bessert, weil er behindert ist? *Die Zeit*, 13 August. Available at: www.zeit.de/2016/33/markus-rehm-olympische-spiele-behinderung-prothese-weitsprung

Howe, P.D. and C. Jones. 2006. Classification of disabled athletes: (dis)empowering the Paralympic practice community. *Sociology of Sport Journal*, 23(1): 29–46.

IPC (International Paralympic Committee). 2017. Classification. Available at: www.paralympic.org/classification

Jespersen, E. and M.J. McNamee. 2008. Philosophy, dis/ability and adapted physical activity. *Sport, Ethics and Philosophy*, 2(2): 86–97.

Jones, C. and P.D. Howe. 2005. The conceptual boundaries of sport for the disabled: classification and athletic performance. *Journal of the Philosophy of Sport*, 32(2): 133–146.

Karpin, I. and R. Mykitiuk. 2008. Going out on a limb: prosthetics, normalcy and disputing the therapy/enhancement distinction. *Medical Law Review*, 16(3): 413–436.

Kram, R., A.M. Grabowski, C.P. McGowan, M.B. Brown and H.M. Herr. 2010. Counterpoint: artificial legs do not make artificially fast running speeds possible. *Journal of Applied Physiology*, 108(4): 1012–1014.

Loland, S. and M. McNamee. 2000. Fair play and the ethos of sports: an eclectic philosophical framework. *Journal of the Philosophy of Sport*, 27(1): 63–80.

Longman, J. 2007. An amputee sprinter: is he disabled, or too abled? *New York Times*, 15 May. Available at: www.nytimes.com/2007/05/15/sports/othersports/15runner.html

Marcellini, A., S. Ferez, D. Issanchou, E. De Léséleuc and M. McNamee. 2012. Challenging human and sporting boundaries: the case of Oscar Pistorius. *Performance Enhancement & Health*, 1(1): 3–9.

Moreton, C. 2012. Oscar Pistorius finally runs in games after five-year battle, 4 August. Available at: www.telegraph.co.uk/sport/olympics/athletics/9452280/London-2012-Olympics-Oscar-Pistorius-finally-runs-in-Games-after-five-year-battle.html

Murray, T.H., K.J. Maschke and A.A. Wasunna. 2009. *Performance-enhancing Technologies in Sports: Ethical, Conceptual, and Scientific Issues*. Baltimore, MD: Johns Hopkins University Press.

Oliver, M. 1990. *The Politics of Disablement: A Sociological Approach*. New York: St Martin's Press.

Oliver, M. 1996. *Understanding Disability: From Theory to Practice*. New York: St Martin's Press.

Oliver, M. 2013. The social model of disability: Thirty years on. *Disability & Society*, 28(7): 1024–1026.

Shakespeare, T. 2012. Still a health issue. *Disability and Health Journal*, 5(3): 129–131.

Shakespeare, T. 2013. *Disability Rights and Wrongs Revisited*. Oxon and New York: Routledge.

Shakespeare, T., L.I. Iezzoni and N.E. Groce. 2009. Disability and the training of health professionals. *The Lancet*, 374(9704): 1815–1816.

Skordilis, E.K., F.A. Skafida, N. Chrysagis and N. Nikitaras. 2006. Comparison of sport achievement orientation of male wheelchair basketball athletes with congenital and acquired disabilities. *Perceptual and Motor Skills*, 103(3): 726–732.

Stein, M.A., P.J. Stein, D. Weiss and R. Lang. 2009. Health care and the UN disability rights convention. *The Lancet*, 374(9704): 1796–1798.

Stucki, G., A. Cieza, T. Ewert, N. Kostanjsek, S. Chatterji and T.B. Üstün. 2002. Application of the International Classification of Functioning, Disability and Health (ICF) in clinical practice. *Disability and Rehabilitation*, 24(5): 281–282.

Tamburrini, C. and T. Tännsjö. 2005. The genetic design of a new Amazon. In *Genetic Technology and Sport: Ethical Questions*, eds C. Tamburrini and T. Tännsjö. London and New York: Routledge, pp. 181–198.

Tännsjö, T. 2009. Medical enhancement and the ethos of elite sport. In *Human Enhancement*, eds J. Savulescu and N. Bostrom. Oxford: Oxford University Press, pp. 315–326.

Teetzel, S. 2014. The onus of inclusivity: sport policies and the enforcement of the women's category in sport. *Journal of the Philosophy of Sport*, 41(1): 113–127.

The Lancet. 2009. Disability: beyond the medical model. Available at: www.thelancet.com/article/S0140-6736(09)62043-2/abstract

Tweedy, S.M. and Y.C. Vanlandewijck. 2011. International Paralympic Committee position stand – background and scientific principles of classification in Paralympic sport. *British Journal of Sports Medicine*, 45(4): 259–269.

UN. 2001. *Convention on the Rights of Persons with Disabilities.* Available at: www.un.org/development/desa/disabilities/convention-on-the-rights-of-persons-with-disabilities.html

Üstün, T.B., S. Chatterji, J. Bickenbach, N. Kostanjsek and M. Schneider. 2003. The International Classification of Functioning, Disability and Health: A new tool for understanding disability and health. *Disability and Rehabilitation*, 25(11–12): 565–571.

Wolbring, G. 2008. The politics of ableism. *Development*, 51(2): 252–258.

Wolbring, G. 2012. Paralympians outperforming Olympians: an increasing challenge for Olympism and the Paralympic and Olympic movement. *Sport, Ethics and Philosophy*, 6(2): 251–266.

10

THE RE-INSCRIPTION OF THE CONCEPT OF BIOLOGICAL RACE THROUGH SPORT IN SOCIETY

10.1. Introduction

Much of the second half of the book has focused on issues of therapy, enhancement and normality, and how these critical concepts in genetics and broader bioethics have played regulatory functions in sport policy and practice. Recent discussions of the genetic basis of sports performance have exacerbated racialised discourses, although many racial assumptions remain problematically covert. In this chapter we explain how the use of the concept of 'human race' is not helpful at either an ontological or at an epistemological level. We then proceed to spell out the ethical implications of the continued use of the concept of race in sport. We conclude that it should be dropped altogether from genetic research, including in the context of sports and sports genetic discussions.

Debates concerning the geneticisation of race reach to social practices beyond sport. Indeed, that reach is global. Debates about the pros and cons of racialised genetics are not just ethical ones, they are also deeply political, being bound up with other embedded social and medical assumptions about normality and abnormality. Although these are not new observations, a more recent twist has arisen in the wake of – or against a background of – the science of 'genetics of sport performance', which offers 'new fertile ground' (Gould 1996) for deeply problematic ideas about the ontological existence of distinct races in the human species. In this chapter we critically analyse how genetics has become the latest tool for the re-inscription and perpetuation of a racial discourse of sport, where it is regrettably seen as ethically unproblematic. We also aim to engage with both an ontological claim ('do human races exist?'); and with an epistemological claim ('can the concept of race be a useful heuristic in genomics research?'), which are not usually the focus of a theoretical engagement in the sociology or philosophy of sport. In addition, we aim to show that there are significant ethical consequences arising from the re-inscription of race through genetics, both in sport and outside sport.

We begin our discussion with some familiar examples from the Olympic Games. Every time there is an Olympics event on television, commentators can scarcely refrain from remarking on the 'fact' that only east African athletes win the long-distance competitions; or that only Asians with their delicate skills excel in the (non-tennis) racket sports; or that only white athletes compete in swimming events. The subtext here is that there must be a biological basis to such prevalence or dominance.

10.2 Black athletes 'just do it better'?

One fairly widely shared assumption is that sports is a cultural space which – given the vast numbers of elite black athletes we see on television – is not discriminatory with regard to matters of race. Thus Hughey and Goss write: 'For many, sports represents the ultimate color blind space [and] as an activity [starting from the Olympics first and foremost] that promotes racial harmony among both participants and observers' (Hughey and Goss 2015, 186). Unfortunately, such a claim is overly simplistic, and neglectful of the inherent deep politicisation of sport throughout history. Immediately prior to the 2012 London Olympic men's 100 metres final, UK's Channel 4 broadcast a BBC-produced documentary titled *Survival of the Fastest*. The programme combined socio biological explanations with snippets of genetic information primarily to ask the question (and answer positively!) that transatlantic slavery created a selection effect that determined the superiority of black athletes.

The media followed with similar explanations on both sides of the pond. It is important to underline that such narratives (both by the media, but also by scientists) are by no means new, but build on a plethora of 'established assumptions that black athletic success is the product of little more than genetic, predisposed traits' that can be dated back (at least) to the victory of African American boxer Jack Johnson as the heavyweight world champion in 1908 (Hughey and Goss 2015, 183). Johnson's victory in 1910 against previously undefeated heavyweight champion James J. Jeffries, the first of many against white opponents, triggered a reconsideration of the physical superiority of whites. The ensuing tension resulted in the demise of white athletic superiority to black athletic superiority, in exchange for the reaffirmation of the white superiority in all other contexts. The 1930s saw the emergence of a spate of 'scientific' studies influenced by the eugenic movement seeking to discover the reasons for black sporting success (Hoberman 1997). While the accomplishments of white athletes were the result of hard work, those of black athletes came to be understood as 'natural' and 'innate'. It was in the 1930s that sporting success, while previously linked to intellectual and aesthetic supremacy, became definitively an indicator of a 'certain limitation of cognitive development' (Carrington 2010, 80).

Consider also the apocryphal 'Jack Nicklaus syndrome', which is an example of the unconscious, often 'benign', acceptance of differences in sports that is premised upon biology or psychology (or a combination of the two). Thus, in 1994, before

Tiger Woods had established himself as the greatest golfer in a generation, Nicklaus was reported to have argued that African American golfers could not succeed at the highest level of golf because of their muscle structure (Hatfield 1996). Similar statements were made in relation to the scarce number of black athletes in swimming, or the similarly low number of white athletes in elite endurance competition (Stone et al. 1999). Another example of the Jack Nicklaus syndrome was a statement made by Sir Roger Bannister, the first person to break the four-minute mile barrier in 1954, who is reported to have said at a 1955 meeting of the British Association for the Advancement of Science that black sprinters may have certain 'anatomical advantages' that give them an edge in track (Anthony 2000). And of course, it was immortalised in the 1992 film *White Men Can't Jump*, about two basketball hustlers – Woody Harrelson and Wesley Snipes – in a tough Los Angeles suburb.

Sociologists of sport have long described how deeply ingrained in sport cultures stereotypes about racial superiority and inferiority are (Carrington 1998; Cashmore 1982; Davis 1990; Fleming 2001; Stone et al. 1999). In the 1970s, the folk-belief that all blacks inherently possessed different or greater musculature was ratified by sociobiological theory about environment, the struggle for natural selection during slavery and the subsequent emergence of the black athlete as a direct descendant of slaves from the plantations. Baker and Horton (2003) have described the phenomenon of 'stereotype threat' according to which in the US blacks opt in to sports like track and field and basketball while opting out of other sports such as swimming or golf. Along similar lines, Brooks has described how black athletes are also complicit in racialising athletic ability (Brooks 2009). Racialised biases seem to be so engrained in Western culture that even black athletes such as Olympic multiple medallist Michael Johnson, in a 2002 documentary, said that slavery 'has benefited descendants like me – I believe there is a superior athletic gene in us' (Gaines 2012).

> In high school, I wondered whether Micheno and the other children of Jamaican parents who made our team so successful might carry some special speed gene they imported from their tiny island. In college, I had the chance to run against Kenyans, and I wondered whether endurance genes might have travelled with them from East Africa.
>
> *(Epstein 2014, xiii–xiv)*

Post hoc rationalisations of athletic superiority being tracked back to the conditions of slavery seem to be very common. Carrington (2010), for one, has described sport as 'generative' of racial discourse with material effects both within the body and beyond.

These points, and more besides, are well known in the significant race-related literature of sociology of sports. Why go over old ground? One justification is that there is a sense of déjà vu in the new debates of race, eugenics and genetics in sports. Moreover, the field of sport can easily 'slip under the radar' of critical analysis in the public consciousness. Why is that the case? One answer might be that the sports context seems *prima facie* to be less 'ethically' problematic than other con-texts, on the grounds that so many black athletes have clearly excelled there. What could be wrong in the first place with praising the 'genetic superiority' of Jamaican athletes in running faster than white athletes? Not only would it seem to be unpro-blematic, but also, possibly, could seem like a laudable thing to do.

How is it that such superficial and discriminatory views came to be so widely held so late in the twentieth century? Part of the answer here is historical and social. Since the early manifestations of sport as a modern social institution during European colonisation, sport has played a central role in popularising notions concerning biological differences that were thought to place black and white people in absolutely different categories. During the first half of the twentieth century sport became the most powerful form of racial spectacle and 'the modality through which popular racism is lived, embodied and challenged' (Carrington 2010, 72–73) This belief, alas, is still alive and kicking. It can still be found in Entine's 2001 book *Taboo: Why Black Athletes Dominate Sport and Why We're Afraid to Talk About it*; in 2014 in David Epstein's *Sports Gene*, and in Nicholas Wade's 2015 book *A Troublesome Inheritance: Race, Genes and Human History*, as we discuss in the next section.

10.3 Old racialised discourses in new clothes

American journalist David Epstein's book *The Sports Gene*, published in 2013 in hard-back, in 2014 in paperback (we refer in this chapter to the paperback edition, with a new and extended foreword), investigates the genetic basis of sport excellence, and is informed by the latest research on the genetic basis of sport performance. Epstein travelled all over the world to speak to athletes and scientists. The book received positive reviews in different outlets on both sides of the Atlantic, such as the *New York Times* and the *Guardian*:[1] people like a good story (especially a story of difficulties and hardships being overcome, as the stories of many athletes are), and Epstein is very good at providing that. The book was hailed as an exemplar of journalistic work that brings together research on the ground (interviews with athletes) and interviews with experts. Despite the title of this book, Epstein is careful not to discount the contributions of environment to athletic excellence, along with other contributions from access to training and coaches as a causal factor for athletic success in American sport. For example, he writes: 'It would be blind and silly to ignore the importance of access to equipment and coaching' (Epstein 2014, 141). But, he also adds:

> This is a book about genetics and athleticism, and it would be just as blind to ignore the conspicuously thorough dominance of people with particular geo-graphic ancestry in certain sports that are globally contested and have few barriers to entry. Namely, of course, that the athletes who are the fleetest of foot, in both short and long distances, are black.

> *(ibid., 141)*

In eliding ancestry/race/ethnicity, Epstein perpetuates the 'myth' of race, which as aptly put by British-American anthropologist Ashley Montagu in his 1942 work *Man's Most Dangerous Myth: The Fallacy of Race* 'is almost impervious to rational thought' (Montagu 1997 (1942), 42).

In his chapter 10, for example, Epstein includes a horrific demonstration of socio-biological theory where he describes the 'warrior-slave theory of Jamaican sprinting'. Apparently the province of Trelawny (Jamaican's north-west), was in the eighteenth century the home to a 'small band of unlikely warriors who descended the sheer limestone cliffs from the thickly layered rain forest of Jamaica's cockpit country into the valleys below to terrorize the most refined soldiers of the world's most feared military' (Epstein 2014, 162). The reader, it seems, is left to make the rather remarkable deduction that this should be enough to explain African American superiority in sport. The book is also ripe with examples of anthropometric biases, which would excite any fan of Lombroso's hypothesis of inherited criminality. To take one example:

> Studies of Olympic athletes are uniformly consistent in finding that Africans and African Americans and African Canadians and Afro-Caribbeans have a more 'linear' build than their competitors of Asian and European descent. That is, they tend to have longer legs and more narrow pelvic breadth.
>
> *(Epstein 2014, 138)*

or another:

> Both white and black players in the NBA have wingspan to height ratios much greater that the population average, but there's a sizeable gap between white and black players.
>
> *(ibid., 139)*

Or yet another:

> There are, however, certain body type differences that have persisted over time and that have attracted the interest of sports anthropometrists. Every study that has examined race differences in body types has documented a disparity between black and white people that remains whether they reside in Africa, Europe, or the Americas. For any given sitting height – that is, the height of one's head when one is sitting in a chair – Africans or African Americans have longer legs than European.
>
> *(ibid., 138)*

The horror continues when Epstein writes about 'Allen's rule' (from American zoologist Joel Asaph Allen who apparently published a 'seminal paper' in 1877):

> The African elephants, having evolved closer to the equator, have developed larger ears for cooling purposes. "Allen's rule", that animals from warmer

climates tend to have longer limbs, has been extended to human by veritable filing cabinet full of studies.

(ibid., 140)

This filing cabinet may be full, but it has been disproved by studies of evolutionary biologist S.J. Gould (Gould 1996) and by Lewontin and others cited below. Relying on arguments from authority is always a precarious matter for both philosophers and scientists.

In Nicholas Wade's 2015 book *A Troublesome Inheritance*, we find yet more examples of sociobiological explanations for the excellence of black athletes. In his book, Wade affirms that race is 'real' and that Darwinian natural selection has resulted in a number of biologically separate human populations characterised by distinct, genetically determined social behaviours in recent time. Yet, as we shall go on to argue, such claims rest on false ontological and epistemological assumptions.

One reason for caution is that the step from praising blacks for their superior athletic traits to the assumption that whites are superior in non-athletic activities can be a very short one. As pointed out by Adesioye, 'If it's OK to equate black dominance in sprinting to biological factors based on race, it also then paves the way for equating black underachievement in education, for example, to inherent racially orientated biological differences, such as smaller brains' (Adesioye 2008). Unfortunately, as noted also by others, among whom John Hoberman is prominent, it is easy to slide from seemingly benign statements that are complimentary to black athletes regarding excellent performances in sport, to racist assumptions about (e.g.) their intellectual inferiority. Hoberman (1997) has noted how the myth of physical supremacy of black athletes is set alongside the rational or strategic superiority of white athletes. More recently, Hughey and Goss (2015) conducted an empirical study to investigate the relationship between the mainstream (English-language) media and essentialist/ biologically determinative assumptions and beliefs about race. After analysing hundreds of newspapers from the United States, UK, South Africa, Canada and Australia, they conclude that 'mainstream media narratives construct and reinforce varied under-standings of race, racial essentialism, genomics, and racialist, if not racist, understandings of the intersection of race and athleticism'. As put by Greg Laden in his review of Wade's book '*A Troublesome Inheritance* is itself troubling, not for its politics, but for its science. Its arguments are only mildly amended versions of arguments discarded decades ago by those who methodically and systematically study human behavioral variation across cultures' (Laden 2016) What is more worrying is that Wade proclaims – and we take his word in good faith – to have written an 'apolitical' book. Going back to the beginning of this chapter, he is not the only one claiming we live in a 'post-racial' world of sport. However, such a view is at best naïve and at worst pernicious and subtle. As Marks (2014, 222) puts it in his review of the book, 'the study of human variation is never just biology; it is, and has always been, biopolitics'. The complete lack of awareness of his-torical context, and of the history of ideas, in Wade and Epstein is culpable. And it is not merely history that this scientific tirade is remiss with: the claim that modern statistical analysis of human genetic variations have revealed a division of our gene pool ignores the work of Lewontin in 1972, Cavalli-Sforza 25 years later, and Barbujani in the early 2000s, that have demonstrated that there is no such subdivision. Both books are prime examples of a long tradition of rationalisations seemingly rooted in biology and in nature masking explanations for social inequalities.

10.4 The Human Genome Project and the predicted demise – turned re-inscription – of race through genomics

The White House ceremony of June 2000 announcing the completion of the draft sequence of the human genome by Francis Collins (National Institutes of Health) and Craig Venter (Celera Genomics) with the then US President Bill Clinton seemed to offer some grounds for hope that the discussion on human race was put to rest. At that ceremony, Craig Venter announced to the whole world that 'The concept of race has no genetic or scientific basis' (Yudell 2014). Collins echoed shortly thereafter with similar remarks. These statements were based on conclusions from the completion of the Human Genome Project which had unequivocally showed that the genetic differences within a population were much higher than the genetic differences between populations. However, things did not turn out quite that way. Was it over-optimism, excessive confidence or just wishful thinking? To understand why genomics did not fulfil its promise of eliminating race from the scientific discourse, we need first a brief digression into genomics research in the last 40 years.

Early scientists trying to list the human races have never been able to reach an agreement, and catalogues proposed since the eighteenth century contain anything between two and 200 races (Barbujani 2005; Barbujani and Pigliucci 2013). Theodosius Dobzhansky (1900–1975), considered the father of evolutionary biology (whose most famous remark was that 'Nothing makes sense if not in the light of evolution'), admitted that human races are poorly defined (epistemological claim), although he maintained that they existed (ontological claim). Dobzhansky predicted (only later to be disproven) evolutionary claims would be better described in the future with the help of genetics tools. By contrast, the geneticist Richard Lewontin (1929–) was adamant that neither the ontological nor the epistemological claim about human races held water. Lewontin is author of a very famous study in 1972 published in *Evolutionary Biology*, where for the first time he showed that populations were more genetically diverse than previously thought, as most genetic variation is contained within populations rather than between populations (85.4% against 8.3%) (Lewontin 1972). From this it follows that most of the variability between human beings can be explained in terms of differences within a population (however defined), not between populations. To put the numbers of his article into words, Lewontin famously remarked: 'If the holocaust comes and a small tribe deep in the New Guinea forests are the only survivors, almost all the genetic variation now expressed among the innumerable groups of our five billion people will be preserved' (cited in Gould 1996, 355). The 1972 article firmly rejected human racial classification on both the biological and social levels, and called for the abandonment of the use of the term race in the human species. Many more of these calls would follow over the ensuing decades. In summary, Lewontin wrote that human racial classification had 'no social value' and 'virtually no genetic or taxonomic significance' (Lewontin 1972, 391). The significance of Lewontin's findings is enhanced when understood within the cultural context of the US at that time (the 1970s and 1980s), where there was turf war with sociobiologists. Lewontin and his mentor S.J. Gould were often engaged directly with Edward O. Wilson, author of *Sociobiology*. Indeed, Lewontin's 1996 book *Biology as Ideology* was a direct response to Wilson's idea, aimed at the explanation of human behaviours on the basis of biology.

To be fair to sociobiologists, not all of them proclaimed the racial inferiority of certain groups: they 'only' predicted that every racial group would be xenophobic, but made no statements about the superiority of some racial groups (at least this was the case for the father of sociobiology, E.O. Wilson). Nevertheless, by finding evolutionary and genetic explanations for why people are racist, they provided a framework to naturalise racism, effectively offering a 'genetic rationale for it' (Yudell 2014, 200). Contrary to sociobiological explanations, the modern synthesis of evolutionary biology teaches us that not all our traits are the products of evolution. Quite on the contrary, most of these traits are the product of contingencies and serve now a function for which they were not actively selected. In technical terms, they are 'exaptations' (Gould and Lewontin 1979).

Twenty-five years after the publication of Lewontin's article, his findings were confirmed by another very famous article spearheaded by Nobel-prize winning geneticist Luca Cavalli-Sforza (1922–). The title of the article, published in the *Proceedings of the National Academy of Science* in 1997 bore – not coincidentally – a striking similarity to Lewontin's 1972 paper: 'An apportionment of human DNA diversity' (Barbujani et al. 1997). The article confirmed Lewontin's thesis and showed that there was no significant genetic discontinuity between any so-called racial groups that would provide a biological basis for any racial classification in the human species – hence disproving the predictions of those, e.g. Dobzhansky, that new genetic tools would eventually be able to classify human races. The study concluded that 'the burden of proof is now on the supporters of a biological basis for human racial classification' (Barbujani et al. 1997, 4519).

Despite Venter's and Collins's public statements about the 'death' of the concept of race, its continued existence in biomedical research shows that its demise had been wishful thinking. Another 20 years have gone by and the burden of proof still seems to be on those who hold – with the latest genetic tool around the block – that the human species cannot be, contrary to Barbujani's prediction, classified into race. In the face of genetic science, writes sociologist Troy Duster, the post-genomics age has witnessed a 'surprising' re-inscription of racial discourse: 'There is substantial evidence that developments in several fields of inquiry and practice related to molecular genetics (pharmacogenomics, pharmacotoxicology, clinical genetics, personalized medicine and forensic science) have actually served to re-inscribe race as a biological category' (Duster 2015, 2).

Dorothy Roberts offers a different interpretation, arguing that race and science have intimately coexisted for 300 years. Tracing back to Ashley Montagu's

(1997/1942) understanding of 'race' as a 'myth' impervious to rational thinking, and genetic data notwithstanding, she notes how some 'scientists have reconfigured race without abandoning it': 'What links racial science from one generation to the next is the quest to update the theories and methods for dividing human beings into a handful of groups to provide a biological explanation for their differences' (Roberts 2011, 26).

Yet this does not address why generations of scientists have stuck to the concept of racial groups. Today's scientists claim that their focus on 'genetic clusters' has excised the political aspects of race from their research. Neil Risch bears much of the responsibility for the perpetuation of race concept in the US in the post-genomic age. Risch is the main proponent of the biological concept of race and supporter of 'race medicine'. He argues that race can serve as a useful heuristic to determine differences in treatment responses or disease prevalence. Risch et al. (2002) write that many genetic studies have come to the identical conclusion, that each continent is home to a race, and claim that they could demonstrate the validity of racial self-categorisation 'from an objective perspective'. In fact, they end up defending the status of race for Hispanics, a group composed of people of different origins who have two features in common, being immigrants in the US and speaking Spanish, neither of which has any genetic basis. Following Risch et al.'s example, racial categories are now routinely employed by US medical doctors and scientists, and in community health (Barbujani et al. 2013). What these scientists remarkably fail to acknowledge is that their own acceptance of racial category influences the decision to inscribe genetic clusters into genomics research itself (Roberts 2011). The theory thus becomes a source of its own evidence, irrespective of the problematic nature of both sources, like two drunks holding each other up at the end of a too social evening.

One problem maintaining the re-inscription of race in genomics science seems to be that the US National Institutes of Health (NIH), in an effort to ensure inclusivity and diversity of populations in genomics data, are requiring the use of 'race' in their studies. Importantly, Duster notes how the US is the only country in the world that, as public health policy, does not operate on the assumption of the single standard human (Duster 2005). Having identified some problematic aspects of Boorse's biostatistical theory of health in Chapter 6, we see here how an attempt at recognising a kind of diversity in genetic science has generated a pernicious differentiation among population groups. Scientists working at, or funded by NIH, are thus mandated to report race based on US Census categories. What this means in practice is that the NIH reifies racial categories in its grant applications. Yudell has referred to this reification as the 'paradox of genomics in the 21st century' (Yudell 2014, 205), where self-reported racial identity remains 'an essential variable used at all stages of genetic research' (ibid.).

Despite these projects' laudable goals of eliminating racisms, it is not through the expansion of supposedly neutral liberal democratic values such as 'participation' or 'inclusion' that racism will be eliminated. On the contrary, what we are seeing is an instance of the 'misplaced concreteness problem' identified by philosopher of science Alfred North Whitehead (1925), as these studies posit the existence of concrete objects where none exist. The objects of the studies are being co-produced as the groups of participants are being created. What can we do to get out of this impasse? Put simply, scholars and policy-makers need to stop considering science a 'neutral' process, and considering the domain of science and the domains of ethics and society as separate:

> It is precisely this understanding of science as a domain apart from base social interests and prejudices – indeed, as a force that might counteract them – that prevents engagement with questions about 'groupness' that lie at the heart of contemporary concerns about human genetic variation research.
>
> *(Reardon 2009, 316)*

And to this we add, the understanding of the genetic basis of sport performance. Leaving the ontological question about human races only to scientists protects their methods of investigation from external scrutiny, and fails to alert policy-makers to the normative choices that are made or assumed but not articulated nor justified explicitly by scientists. One implication of this recognition is again a renewed demand for multidisciplinary scholarship in the bioethics of sports. Moreover, not only is philosophical work in medicine and sport essential, as we have seen, but we need to draw on work in the philosophy of biology too.

10.5 The future is now: whole genome sequencing and the epistemic disutility of the concept of race

Lewontin, writing in 1972, and Barbujani and Cavalli-Sforza, writing 25 years later in 1997, made the point that the 'burden of proof' to demonstrate the genetic basis of race was on those who believed there is such a basis. They also pointed to future whole genome sequencing studies that may confirm their data about the higher level of genetic variability within rather than between populations. Another 20 years have gone by, and with the sequencing of a greater number of human genomes and the completion of the Human Genome Diversity Project that future predicted by Lewontin and Barbujani and Cavalli-Sforza is now here. What has that future brought? Scientists have not been able to unequivocally define races with the help of new genetic tools; on the contrary, as pointed out by philosopher of biology Lorusso (2011), different racial clusters identified with high-power statistical modelling have failed to cross-validate.

The biological evidence we have gathered from whole genome sequencing studies has confirmed previous data by Lewontin (1972) and Barbujani et al. (1997), among others, that the distribution of different genetic traits is consistently continuous across populations in the human species. Put differently, discontinuity in genetic traits (a logically necessary condition for the existence of races) is not supported by biological evidence. In the human species, there are no discontinuities, except for rare cases of single traits in extreme situations of populations that have been isolated for a long time, and that anyway do not correspond to any racial cluster.

In a good although too rare example of an intellectual collaboration between a scientist and a philosopher population geneticist Barbujani and philosopher of science Pigliucci have argued that

> The analysis of large genomic datasets is showing why it proved impossible to find an agreement on the main biological groups of humankind. Among nearly 250,000 polymorphic genome sites, no single-nucleotide polymorphism was found at which a fixed difference would distinguish any pair of continental populations.
>
> *(Barbujani and Pigliucci 2013, 137)*

From this we can draw two conclusions, namely: (i) any classification on the basis of the genetic properties in the human species is totally arbitrary from a biological point of view; and (ii) even if genetic clusters could be created from statistically significant boundaries, these would not be unambiguous, and they would still not be projectable, nor could they be used reliably as heuristic tools. This discussion is – obviously – not a relevant issue only for philosophers, social scientists or bioethicists; it also has tremendously important repercussions in the medico-scientific community. Notwithstanding what some scientists such as Risch or Collins may assert regarding the instrumental value of using the concept of race in biomedical research, the idea of developing different drugs for a specific disease for different human clusters depends on the following three ontological assumptions of which (1) and (2) are necessary but not sufficient for (3) to obtain:

1. that races exist (that genetic discontinuities exist among populations within human species);
2. that there is a genetic basis for the disease that is being analysed; and
3. that differences in disease rates among racial clusters are causally related to genetic discontinuities among racial clusters.

It goes without saying that *it would not make sense* to develop racially targeted drugs if we knew that either premise (1) or premise (2) were false. What we do know is that premise (2) is true. However, whole genome sequencing data have demonstrated that premise (1) is false. Consequently, it does not make sense to develop drugs specific for one racial cluster, since we know that the trait is continuously distributed across racial clusters, and the racial cluster cannot be used as a heuristic for the prediction of the frequency of traits. Lorusso concludes that 'A racial cluster does not necessarily carry any genetic information that can be used in biomedical research in order to make predictions' (Lorusso 2011, 538). In other words, *the concept of race has no independently testable consequences in medicine, and when it is introduced in biomedical research, it is introduced 'ad hoc'*. The best way to find out whether a person is a normal (statistically speaking), slow or fast metaboliser is to study that person's DNA, not try to infer that information from some characteristics of a group to which we have ascribed that person to. To predict an individual response to a drug, we need to look at individual genomes (Barbujani 2005, 8). We now turn to the implications for genetics in sports that attempt to consider racial groups as objects of targeted interventions or personalised sports medicine.

10.6 Ethical and social implications of the re-inscription of race in the genetic basis of sport performance

Sporting contests today are rarely seen as explicitly embodying racial meaning. While some say that sports today signal the actualisation of some kind of 'post-racial settlement' where race no longer matters, we are less optimistic and more inclined to agree with Carrington's (2010) critical analysis. According to Carrington, the fact that ideas about race have changed and shifted does not mean that racism itself, and the racialised cultural structures related to it, have disappeared from the sport scene. Carrington argues for a non-individualistic conception of racist structures that enable us to see 'how racist effects can be produced without the need for "racist intent" and that scholars pay more attention to sport as a critical site for the reproduction and re-articulation of forms of racial knowledge' (Carrington 2010, 174).

Importantly, Epstein and Wade completely overlook the consequences of the reification of race through studies on the genetic basis of sport performance: a vicious circle is created. Racially self-identified groups are asked to participate on the wrong premise that these groups are based on ontological categories based in nature/science, and the results are used to reinforce such social categories. One tangible consequence noted above is that athletes will not participate in sports that they think are not suitable for them, actualising what is known as 'stereotype threat'. Another problematic ethical consequence of the genetically renewed discourse of race in sport can be captured by the following hypothetical, although plausible, scenario: if only we were able to know what genetically distinguished an elite distance runner from an elite sprint runner early on, we would be able to *intervene early* in the process of selecting and producing such champions. This, as the reader might recognise it, would be a classic example of an early intervention the kind of which we criticised heavily in Chapter 3. Yet it is not only witnessed in sports; other notable examples can be found, for example, in psychiatry, through the search of genetic biomarkers which would allow us to intervene – and treat – early before the onset of the disorder (McGlashan 2001; Singh and Rose 2009). And within the field of bioethics, Julian Savulescu has written in several instances about the 'the ethics of gifted genes' (Savulescu and Foddy 2007; Savulescu 2009; Savulescu 2015). In his most recent article (2015) on the subject, he writes: 'Recent research out of the UK has identified a genetic 'general academic achievement factor'. Using identical twin studies, it is claimed that achievement across a wide range of academic subjects was influenced by many of the same genes: 'genes explain a larger proportion of the differences between children across different subjects (54–65%) than shared environmental factors, such as home and school environment combined (14–21%).' Savulescu takes these data to mean that 'Academic giftedness […] is largely genetic'. Of course extrapolating from single studies is a dangerous game. However, as highlighted in Chapter 1, we are never justified in inferring from the mere fact that a trait is heritable that it is genetically determined. Errors of reductionism and bio-determinism occur in statements such as 'intelligence is 60% genetic and 40% environmental', or 'scientists have found that athletic excellence is … % genetic and % environmental' and so on. Heritability is not a measure of 'how genetic' a trait is, but it is a technical notion which refers to the 'the proportion of the phenotypic variation in a trait of interest, measured in a given studied population and in a given environment, that is statistically co-varying with genetic differences (however measured) among individuals in the same population' (Kaplan 2015). For heritability to make any sense at all as a statistic, the trait in question must vary within the population in question (ibid.). Certainly, we cannot expect the public to be able to navigate such technical notions, and to be fair to Savulescu, as a philosopher and bioethicist, he is not primarily responsible for the representation of genetic findings – scientists are responsible in the first place here and the media in second. Nevertheless, as scholars, we believe we are responsible for uncritical representation of data or selective misrepresentation in our arguments. Understanding the science critically, and presenting it thus, is a responsibility for bioethicists. Good bioethics needs to be informed by a good and critical understanding of biology, and by a good critical understanding of philosophy of biology (Lewens 2015). And in genetics, as in every other branch of science, the facts never speak for themselves (Midgley 2002). Nor is this a hidden claim for philosophical neutrality, just a call for due caution with the data and its power, perceived or otherwise.

American philosopher of biology and bioethicist James Tabery is an example of a scholar who takes that responsibility seriously, and questions the ethical and social implications of early interventions in genetics, in the context of child-rearing. He observes that a trait can be heritable and at the same time completely malleable, and 'when causative factors interact so complexly, and throughout growth to produce an intricate adult being, we cannot, in principle, parse that being's behaviour into quantitative percentages of remote root causes' (Tabery 2014, 34). While several scholars[2] have analysed the ethical implications of genetic testing in children in terms of a possible breach of a 'right to an open future', Tabery goes one step further and describes how genetic knowledge that provides us with information about genetic susceptibilities, i.e. interactions between genes and a particular environment, could lead to a change in the meaning of parenting responsibilities.

Think about a possible scenario: suppose that we had the genetic knowledge to know that we could intervene in a child's environment to the point that this will impact on some interactional traits that the child has, and this in turn will make a difference on whether some of the child's 'susceptibilities' will be actualised in the future. What are the consequences of this knowledge for parental responsibility? Tabery asks, as both a parent and a philosopher, ought we not to 'intervene' in a child's environment if and where it is in their best interests? Yet he notes the subtle difference between two interpretations: on the one hand we might think responsible parenting is helping to shape the life of a child according to their emerging predispositions and talents, and a more or less informed view of the traps to be avoided; while in the other we may be driving crucial child-rearing decisions by a 'duty' to act on the basis of genetic knowledge. Given what we know about the under-determination of genetics in terms of complex traits, this would seem not an enlightened scientifically informed path, but a rather submissive bowing down to the latest genetic meta-analysis. Basing a principle of procreative beneficence on a flawed understanding of the meaning of genetic inheritance is hardly parental progress.

Parenting, like all forms of child and youth development – including sports of course too – is about making decisions in the thick of things. We saw in Chapter 3 how there was no place at which one could step out of the living of a life and make a decision about how best to go forward. A crucial part of that critical reflection in the midst of things is a careful attention to the language in which options are expressed, supported, denigrated and so on. And this is especially the case in matters of race, sports and the latest pseudo-scientific extrapolation of genetically inspired racism. As Yudell puts it, 'the scientific language of race has a significant influence on how the public (which includes scientists) understands human diversity' (Yudell et al. 2016, 565).

Sports scholars and coaches and policy-makers, no less than bioethicists, need to be wary of the latest reincarnation of old ideas of biologically determined inequalities. More than 30 years ago in his book *The Mismeasure of Man* (Gould 1996), evolutionary biologist Stephen Jay Gould cautioned against the dangers of biological explanations for social inequalities. There he re-analysed primary data from Cyril Burt's famous twin studies and Lombroso's before him, and demonstrated how – one by one – measurements and reifications of intelligence fell under the hammer of biases and deeply engrained racial biases. The latest of such reincarnations is through genetics, which is – conveniently – used to explain away social differences, and provide flawed evidence to take away money from educational programmes aimed at redressing such inequalities.

Gould's book was first published in 1981. In the second expanded and revised edition in 1996, he warned specifically against the 'particular appeal of genetic explanations'. More recently, population geneticist Barbujani, cited above, wrote, echoing Gould: 'We should all be aware that the persistence of a racial paradigm in some sectors of research and medical practice guarantees that man will continue to be mismeasured, and that prejudice will keep finding pseudoscientific justifications' (Barbujani et al. 2013, 142).

This is why journalistic, or academic, efforts to racialise sporting excellence on genetic grounds must be challenged before they gather further momentum.

10.7 Conclusions

Returning to the two levels of investigations cited earlier in this chapter, we can conclude: (i) at the ontological level races in the human species do not exist and

(ii) at the epistemological level races are not only *not* 'needed' in biomedical research, but they are not even helpful. They cannot be used as heuristics to predict differences in rates of diseases among populations. Their continued use in biomedical research is unwarranted and may have very serious consequences for the individual, in addition to having negative social consequences by re-inscribing racial stereotypes in society.

Yudell et al. call for a phasing out of racial terminology in biological studies. They write that the concept is 'problematic at best and harmful at worst [and that] it is time for biologists to find a better way' to describe genetic diversity (Yudell et al. 2016, 564). They go on to suggest that scientific journals and professional societies use terms like 'ancestry' or 'populations' to describe human groupings in genetic studies and, most importantly, call on scholars and scientists more clearly to define how they use these variables.

We firmly agree with Yudell et al. and believe that scientists, philosophers and bioethicists have a responsibility to abandon these terms if they cannot be used correctly, and they cannot. Importantly, philosophers have a moral duty to engage with the ontological and epistemological questions around race, as we should not leave unscrutinised the assumptions used by scientists and underlying large genomics research. While we should be wary of castigating wolves in sheep's clothing, the perception of genetic exceptionalism will too easily find a home in sports discourses, and history has taught us that discrimination against historically subjugated populations will all too readily denigrate them further. As philosophers of both medicine and sport we have a duty to question genetic and other medico-scientific narratives that explain human differences away, and to reject flawed assumptions underlying genomics research and any racialised genetics of sport performance.

Notes

All websites accessed October 2017.

1 www.theguardian.com/books/2013/aug/22/sports-gene-david-epstein-review; www.nytimes.com/2013/08/13/science/the-sports-gene-considers-the-root-of-athletic-success.html
2 Including one of us, Camporesi (in Camporesi 2013).

References

All websites accessed October 2017.

Adesioye, L. 2008. Is race a factor in sports success? *Guardian*, 25 August. Available at: www.theguardian.com/commentisfree/2008/aug/25/race.olympics2008

Anthony, A. 2000. White men can't run. *Guardian*, 4 June. Available at: www.theguardian.com/observer/osm/story/0,,328508,00.html

Baker, J. and S. Horton. 2003. East African running dominance revisited: a role for stereotype threat? *British Journal of Sports Medicine*, 37(6): 553–555.

Barbujani, G. 2005. Human races: classifying people vs understanding diversity. *Current Genomics*, 6(4): 215–226.

Barbujani, G. and M. Pigliucci. 2013. Human races. *Current Biology*, 23(5): R185–R187.

Barbujani, G., S. Ghirotto and F. Tassi. 2013. Nine things to remember about human genome diversity. *HLA*, 82(3): 155–164.

Barbujani, G., A. Magagni, E. Minc and L. Cavalli-Sforza. 1997. An apportionment of human DNA diversity. *Proceedings of the National Academy of Sciences*, 94(9): 4516–4519.

Brooks, S.N. 2009. *Black Men Can't Shoot*. Chicago: University of Chicago Press.

Camporesi, S. 2013. Bend it like Beckham! The ethics of genetically testing children for athletic potential. *Sport, Ethics and Philosophy*, 7(2): 175–185.

Carrington, B. 1998. Sport, masculinity, and black cultural resistance. *Journal of Sport and Social Issues*, 22(3): 275–298.

Carrington, B. 2010. *Race, Sport and Politics: The Sporting Black Diaspora*. London: Sage.

Cashmore, E. 1982. *Black Sportsmen*. London and New York: Routledge and Kegan Paul.

Davis, L.R. 1990. The articulation of difference: White preoccupation with the question of racially linked genetic differences among athletes. *Sociology of Sport Journal*, 7(2): 179–187.

Duster, T. 2005. Race and reification in science. *Science*, 307(5712): 1050–1051.

Duster, T. 2015. A post-genomic surprise. The molecular reinscription of race in science, law and medicine. *The British Journal of Sociology*, 66(1): 1–27.

Entine, J. 2001. *Taboo: Why Black Athletes Dominate Sports and Why We're Afraid to Talk About It*. New York: Public Affairs.

Epstein, D.J. 2014. *The Sports Gene: What Makes the Perfect Athlete*. New York: Penguin.

Fleming, S. 2001. Racial science and South Asian and Black physicality. In *Race, Sport and British Society*, eds B. Carrington and I. McDonald. London: Routledge, pp. 105–120.

Gaines, C. 2012. Gold medalist believes descendants of slaves will dominate Olympics thanks to a 'superior athlete gene'. *Business Inside*, 5 July. Available at: www.busi nessinsider.com/gold-medalist-michael-johnson-believes-descendants-of-slaves-will-dom inate-olympics-because-of-a-superior-athlete-gene-2012-7?IR=T

Gould, S.J. 1996. *The Mismeasure of Man*. New York: W.W. Norton & Company.

Gould, S.J. and R.C. Lewontin. 1979. The spandrels of San Marco and the Panglossian paradigm: a critique of the adaptationist programme. *Proceedings of the Royal Society of London B: Biological Sciences*, 205(1161): 581–598.

Hatfield, D. 1996. The Jack Nicklaus syndrome. *Humanist*, 56(4): 38–39.

Hoberman, J.M. 1997. *Darwin's Athletes: How Sport Has Damaged Black America and Preserved the Myth of Race*. New York: Houghton Mifflin Harcourt.

Hughey, M.W. and D.R. Goss. 2015. A level playing field? Media constructions of athletics, genetics, and race. *ANNALS of the American Academy of Political and Social Science*, 661(1): 182–211.

Kaplan, J.M. 2015. Heritability: a handy guide. *Scientia Salon*, 1 June. Available at: https:// scientiasalon.wordpress.com/2015/06/01/heritability-a-handy-guide-to-what-it-means- what-it-doesnt-mean-and-that-giant-meta-analysis-of-twin-studies/

Laden, G. 2016. A troubling tome. *American Scientist*. Available at: www.americanscientist. org/bookshelf/id.16216,content.true,css.print/bookshelf.aspx

Lewens, T. 2015. *The Biological Foundations of Bioethics*. Oxford: Oxford University Press.

Lewontin, R.C. 1972. The apportionment of human diversity. In *Evolutionary Biology*, eds T. Dobzhansky, M.K. Hecht and W.C. Steere. New York: Springer, pp. 381–398.

Lewontin, R. 1996. *Biology as Ideology: The Doctrine of DNA*. New York: Harper Collins.

Lorusso, L. 2011. The justification of race in biological explanation. *Journal of Medical Ethics*, 37(9): 535–539.

McGlashan, T.H. 2001. Psychosis treatment prior to psychosis onset: ethical issues. *Schizophrenia Research*, 51(1): 47–54.

Marks, J. 2014. Review of *A Troublesome Inheritance* by Nicholas Wade. *Human Biology*, 86(3): 221–226.

Midgley, M. 2002. *Wisdom, Information and Wonder: What Is Knowledge for?* Abingdon: Routledge.

Montagu, A. 1997 (1942). *Man's Most Dangerous Myth: The Fallacy of Race*. 6th edition. Oxford, UK: AltaMira Press.

Reardon, J. 2009. *Race to the Finish: Identity and Governance in an Age of Genomics*. Princeton, NJ: Princeton University Press.

Risch, N., E. Burchard, E. Ziv and H. Tang. 2002. Categorization of humans in biomedical research: genes, race and disease. *Genome Biology*, 3(7): 1–12.

Roberts, D. 2011. *Fatal Invention: How Science, Politics, and Big Business Re-Create Race in the Twenty-first Century*. New York: The New Press.

Savulescu, J. 2009. Genetic interventions and the ethics of enhancement of human beings. *Read Philosoph of Tech*, 16(1): 417–430.

Savulescu, J. 2015. The ethics of 'gifted' genes: the road to Gattaca? *Australasian Science*, September. Available at: www.australasianscience.com.au/article/issue-september-2015/ethics-gifted-genes-road-gattaca.html

Savulescu, J. and B. Foddy. 2007. To Gattaca and beyond. In *Human Genetics: Ethics & Issues*, 294 (Issues in Society series), pp. 27–28. Thirroul: The Spinney Press. (Reprinted from To Gattaca and beyond, *The Age*, 29 April 2007.)

Singh, I. and N. Rose. 2009. Biomarkers in psychiatry. *Nature*, 460(7252): 202–207.

Stone, J., C.I. Lynch, M. Sjomeling and J.M. Darley. 1999. Stereotype threat effects on Black and White athletic performance. *Journal of Personality and Social Psychology*, 77(6): 1213–1227.

Tabery, J. 2014. *Beyond Versus: The Struggle to Understand the Interaction of Nature and Nurture*. Cambridge, MA: MIT Press.

Wade, N. 2015. *A Troublesome Inheritance: Genes, Race and Human History*. New York: Penguin.

Whitehead, Alfred North. 1925. *Science and the Modern World*. Cambridge: Cambridge University Press.

Yudell, M. 2014. *Race Unmasked: Biology and Race in the Twentieth Century*. New York: Columbia University Press.

Yudell, M., D. Roberts, R. DeSalle and S. Tishkoff. 2016. Taking race out of human genetics. *Science*, 351(6273): 564–565.

EPILOGUE

This book is the product of a collaboration over seven years, spanning different topics in the ethics and philosophy of sport. Our shared interests in the discussion of the application of emerging technologies to the context of sport, together with our combined expertise in philosophy, ethics and genetics, have led us to pursue the project of this book, which has been long in coming. At the same time, we share a commitment to a critical scrutiny of the science underlying the new technologies. Part of our methodology is therefore to discuss realistic scenarios grounded in scientific feasibility, and not in science fiction, or long-term scientific guesswork. In addition we have been committed to the contextualisation of the discussions in philosophy of sport, and to an awareness of the historical and political landscapes in which the related issues have arisen. Although starting from two slightly different biopolitical positions (Camporesi more on the bioliberal side, McNamee more on the bioconservative side), we have found common grounds and were able to reach shared positions regarding the discussions arisen in this volume.

As we are writing this epilogue, in August 2017, the US personal genomics company Helix (a spin-off of Illumina) is launching an 'app store' where for 80$ customers can buy interpretations of their DNA in order to create 'a lifelong relationship with their DNA data';[1] IAAF is preparing the appeal to the Court of Arbitration for Sport against the suspension of the Hyperandrogenism Regulations;[2] China is witnessing a boom in commercial genetic testing in an effort to identify early children's talents in a variety of contexts, including dance, mathematics, arts and sports.[3]

Genetics has never been more pervasive in any aspect of our lives, from reproduction, to ageing, to well-being and fitness, to of course, elite sport. Genetic technologies allow us – in varying degrees – to shape ourselves and future generations, raising unique issues at the intersection of autonomy and determination of others, and creating tensions where competing narratives (e.g. individual autonomy versus public health) meet. Through the lens of sport we see re-enacted and re-articulated many of the discussions prompted by genetics in different contexts of life. Because of the unique values that characterise this context, the lens of sport is particularly appropriate to shed new light on some older bioethics questions. Indeed, sport seems to be the context in which some actions that might not be justified elsewhere become justified. On the one hand, think of screening pro-grammes for talent identification and development: although we noted there are strong epistemic challenges with these programmes, there is an appetite of coaches, trainers and parents towards these tests, and also of governments (we noted how China and Uzbekistan have already put in place programmes to identify future champions, in what could be called a well-meaning eugenic effort).[4] Or so they hope.

One might reasonably foresee that as soon as genetics has made the necessary advances with genome-wide association studies, these tests will take off irrespective of the ethical issues identified in Chapter 3. We are under no illusions that the direct to consumer industry will be cowed by ethical arguments. A further example of actions that appear justified in the sport context, although not necessarily in others, is the praising of the athletic potential of some human races or ethnic groups to the detriment of others, with the consequent corollary claims that go with it. On the one hand, as we have shown in Chapter 10, under the guise of praising black athletes for running faster or jumping further, there is a long and perilous tradition of colonialist thinking, and seriously flawed epistemic assumptions about the classification of human beings into racial groups. It is beyond time that we jettisoned this discourse once and for all.

On the other hand, there are actions that may be ethically justified outside the context of sport on grounds of autonomy – taking cognitive enhancing substances for recreation – but that are considered impermissible in sport due to the unique values (of fairness, or level playing field in competition, and – also – of human nature) that characterise it. We are thinking here of therapies that enhance (bios-tatistically derived) normal, or species-typical function and that are impermissible in the light of the global regulatory framework, i.e. the World Anti Doping Code.

Another example that is perhaps uniquely problematic in the context of sport is the mandating of pharmacological modification (testosterone reduction) of certain (hyperandrogenic) women in order to 'normalise' their bodies and have them conform to some heteronormative standard of femininity under the guise of redressing a purported 'level playing field in competition'. While outside the context of sport an increasing number of countries have recognised that sex/gender is not binary, but a continuum, the world of professional sports remains incredibly anachronistic and detached from progressive law making that allow individuals to choose a non-binary gender. Other examples of discontinuities between actions that can be justified in the context of sport but not outside, or vice versa, abound in this volume, and are key to shed a a different light on the biopolitical axis and ramifications of genetics through all our aspects of our life.

This is why, as we argue throughout this book, we need a contextual, case-by-case approach to the ethical evaluation of genetic and other biotechnologies. We have made this point repeatedly in this volume: from the ethical evaluation of gene transfer to raise the tolerance to pain in the elite sport and in the therapeutic context (Chapter 7), to the ethical evaluation of the types of genetic testing offered in sport (Chapter 2), to the evaluation of assistive technologies for Paralympics athletes (Chapter 9), to the evaluation of biobanking projects and whole genome screening projects (Chapter 4). It is sport that allows a re-articulation of norms that may appear over-used elsewhere, such as respect for autonomy, and the therapy/enhancement distinction.

With genome editing technologies such as CRISPR we now have the means to alter future generations and control our own evolution. Questions surrounding its permissibility or desirability of course remain. Leading bioliberal scholars, such as John Harris, have been arguing for years that we should; others, such as the bio-conservative Michael Sandel, are more cautious. Even Jennifer Doudna, one of the two co-discoverers of CRISPR, although being cautious about some of the applications of the technology, envisions a future in which we may be morally culpable if we were not to use CRISPR to screen out diseases or disabilities once we had the safe means to do so. The line between the moral obligation to act, and the moral obligation not to act, is a disputed one. Another important point that we made repeatedly in this volume is the inextricable link between epistemology and ethics, which we made in Chapter 3 in relation to DTC genetic testing, in Chapter 4 in relation to big data and biobanking, and in Chapter 10 in relation to race. This is a point too often obscured by bioethicists who engage cursorily with the scientific claims and proceed to discuss the ethical implications, without troubling themselves – which we argue is the duty of any philosopher – to be informed as to whether such scientific claims stand scrutiny. Good bioethics, and good sports ethics, need to be informed by a critical understanding of science, and – in the case of genetics – a critical understanding of philosophy of biology. Hence, as we observe, at the intersection of bioethics, genetics and sports, there is a pressing need for multidisciplinary scholarship. To engage in the ethical issues which arise from the application of new genetic technologies means also to engage – at least to some extent – with the epistemological issues surrounding genetics e.g. what a gene is, what a gene does; what it means for a trait to be heritable; what it means to classify human beings in groups; what it means for a genotype to be expressed phenotypically, and so on and so forth.

The future of sport may be said to lie at the intersection of two trajectories: the geneticisation of the athlete, and the hyperbolic 'cyborgysation' of the athlete. These two axes intersect and raise fundamental questions about the significance of human nature, as already identified by Hoberman (1992) more than 25 years ago, which are core questions in bioethics and sports ethics writ large. Genetics and biomechanics raise unique questions about the role, and value, of technology in sport. What will our Olympic athlete in 30, or 50, years look like? The answer to that question depends on the answer to the question of how our average 'human' will look like. Genetically modified? Cyborg? A bit of both? Exciting, some say. Scary, perhaps terrifying, others reply. Future gazing is a precarious occupation. Nevertheless, sticking our heads in the sand and pretending that these changes are not happening, or may not happen, is not a meritorious response. We know from sports advances that once the technology is available, it will be used. The genie cannot be put back into the bottle. Ethical estimations and evaluations of the science and genetic future of sports medicine should be a driver to react critically, to tackle head-on difficult questions that will shape our conceptions not simply of sports or athletes, but of the human condition itself.

Notes

All websites accessed October 2017.

1 www.genomeweb.com/scan/helix-launches-app-store
2 www.hindustantimes.com/other-sports/dutee-chand-s-gender-case-to-be-re-opened-iaaf-to-return-to-cas/story-vqQ77jYyIECGaJkIksiVTI.html
3 www.telegraph.co.uk/news/2017/02/11/anxious-chinese-parents-fuel-gene-testing-boom-try-discover/
4 www.theatlantic.com/international/archive/2014/02/uzbekistan-is-using-genetic-testing-to-find-future-olympians/283001/;   www.telegraph.co.uk/news/2017/02/11/anxious-chinese-parents-fuel-gene-testing-boom-try-discover/

References

Hoberman, J. 1992. *Mortal Engines. The Science of Performance and the Dehumanization of Sport.* New York: The Free Press.

GLOSSARY

Allele/alleles   Each gene can occur in several possible forms, known as 'alleles'. In human beings, there typically are two alleles for each gene, one of which is located on each chromosome and one of which is inherited from each parent.

Aneuploid   A cell is said to be aneuploid when it contains an abnormal number of chromosomes, for example 45 or 47 instead of the normal 46 for the human species. One common example in the human species is Down Syndrome or trisomy 21, where there are three copies of chromosomes 21, leading to a total number of chromosomes of 47.

Chromosomes   Chromosomes are discrete, compact units of the genome where DNA molecules are organised. Each unit carries from hundreds to thousands of tightly packed genes (chromosomes vary widely in size and number of genes). The human species has 23 pairs of chromosomes (each chromosome of the same pair is called *homologous*), which become unpacked during cellular division.

Cytoplasm   All the material inside the cell and outside the nucleus in eukaryotic cells. It includes different organelles such as *mitochondria*.

DNA   Deoxyribonucleic acid. It is found in all eukaryotic cells' nuclei. It is formed by four different nitrogen bases (adenine (A), thymine (T), cytosine (C) and guanine (G)) that bind in sequence and make a single DNA strand. Each base binds to its complementary base (A to T and C to G) to form a double stranded DNA. In these two strands all the genetic information – the blueprint of the information to codify for life – is included. Each triplet of bases is called a 'codon' and codifies for an amino acid, one of the building blocks of proteins, which are themselves the building blocks of living organisms. During replication the two strands open up and one copies itself to form another complementary strand that contains the same genetic information.

Eukaryotic/prokaryotic   Eukaryotic cells have the genetic material organised into a membrane-bound nucleus which is distinct from the rest of the cell, while prokaryotic cells have no distinction between nucleus and cytoplasm. Prokaryotic cells are bacteria and archaea. Eukaryotic cells build up the rest of the living organisms on Earth!

Euploid   Cells containing a normal number of chromosomes for that species (in the human species, it is 46), or containing two chromosomes for each pair of homologous chromosomes.

Gametes   Gametes, also known as sex cells or germ cells, are found in the gonads, or sexual organs. In the human species they are sperm and oocytes, the latter also known as eggs. Gametes differ from somatic cells insofar as they are *haploid* (they contain half the number of chromosomes than somatic cells, i.e. 23 in the human species). When a gamete cell fuses with another gamete cell of the opposite sex during fertilisation it leads to the production of a zygote.

Gene   Genetics is a matter of genes, of course. However, what is a gene is not such an easy question; on the contrary, it is a philosophical question! One of the most important findings of molecular genetics is that the idea of a gene as a simple causal agent is not valid. The sequence of DNA that is referred to as a 'gene' has meaning only within a specific context, which determines its expression and function. That is why a single gene may have different effects depending on the context in which it is located (cellular context, environmental context, individual context, etc.). For the purposes of this book, a gene is usually considered a specific region of the genome whose DNA sequence encodes for a discrete biological entity, usually a protein. The human genome has about 21,000 genes.

Genome   By 'genome', we refer to the entire genetic material that is transmitted to the next generation. In the human species, it is for the most part encoded in the DNA sequence contained in the nuclei of our cells, although we have a small number of genes in the *mitochondria*, which, if mutated, are responsible for some types of neurodegenerative diseases.

Genotype/phenotype   The term genotype refers to the genetic constitution of an organism, and is commonly found in opposition to phenotype, which refers instead to the appearance of an organism, resulting from the interactions of its genetic constitutions with the environment.

Haploid   A cell is said to be 'haploid' if it contains one of every pair of homologous chromosomes. Gametes are haploid and in the human species contain 23 chromosomes.

Haplotype   'Haplotype' refers to the combination of alleles in a defined region of a chromosome, while 'linkage' refers to the (probabilistic) tendency of genes to be inherited together as a result of their location on the same chromosome; it is measured by the percentage of recombination between genetic loci.

Heritability   Heritability refers to the proportion of the phenotypic variation in a trait of interest, measured in a given studied population and in a given environment. It is defined operationally as the ratio of variation due to differences between genotypes to the total phenotypic variation for a character or trait in a population. Put a bit more simply, heritability refers to the amount of phenotypic (observable) variation in a given population that is attributable to individual genetic differences. Note that for a trait to be 'heritable' does not mean to be genetically fixed or determined, as the expression of the trait will still be influenced by the environmental conditions. That is why a trait can be said to have complete heritability (H=1) but still be altered drastically by environmental changes. An example is the genetic disorder phenylketonuria, which can be treated effectively with diets that avoid the amino acid phenylalanine.

Homologous   Usually refers to chromosomes. Two chromosomes are said to be 'homologous' if they carry the same genetic loci. This doesn't mean that they have the same DNA sequence, as each chromosome may carry a different allele at the same genetic locus. The human species has, normally, 23 pairs of homologous chromosomes, one from each parent.

Homozygous/heterozygous   For each gene, an individual can be homozygous, meaning having two identical alleles, or heterozygous, meaning having two different alleles. Individuals are said to be heterozygous when they have different alleles at a particular locus, and homozygous when they have the same allele at corresponding loci on the homologous chromosome.

Karyotype   With the word 'karyotype' we refer to the entire chromosomal complement of a cell or species, in the case of the human species, 23 pairs, XX for women, XY for men. A karyotypic analysis is typically performed during prenatal screening to establish the absence of chromosomal disorders, of which the most common in the human species is trisomy 21 or Down Syndrome (in which there are three instead of two copies of chromosome 21).

Locus/loci   By 'locus' we refer to the position on a chromosome at which the gene for a particular trait resides. Different alleles occupy the same locus on homologous chromosomes.

Meiosis   Form of specialised cell division happening in sexually reproducing organisms that gives rise to the production of four haploid gametes, each containing one of every pair of homologous chromosomes.

Mitochondria   Organelles contained in all eukaryotic cells' cytoplasm. They have the function to provide energy to the cells, that is why they are often called the 'powerhouses' of the cell. They have their own genome. They codify for 37 genes in the human species. If mutated, these genes can give rise to severe neurodegenerative disorders. Recently a technique has been developed called mitochondrial replacement transfer that is a variation of *in vitro* fertilisation and allows the replacement of the mitochondria carrying the mutation with mitochondria from a third party.

Mitosis   The process by which a eukaryotic somatic cell divides into two daughter cells.

Monogenic vs polygenic   Traits controlled by a single gene are said to be 'monogenic'. In genetics, monogenetic traits are a minority, and result from modifications in a single gene. Most traits are polygenic, meaning they are the result of the effects of many different genes. Common monogenic diseases are cystic fibrosis, thalassaemia, sickle-cell anaemia, Tay-Sachs, fragile X syndrome and Huntington's disease. Monogenic diseases, although rare, affect millions of people worldwide. They are divided in three categories: dominant (a trait that needs to have only one mutated copy of DNA to appear phenotypically), recessive (a trait that needs to have two mutated copies of the gene to appear phenotypically) or X-linked (meaning that the gene causing the trait or the disorder is located on the X chromosome, leading to male/female differences in expressions, as females carrying two copies of the gene usually are healthy carriers of the disorder but do not normally express the symptoms, e.g. Duchenne muscular dystrophy).

Organelle   Literally, 'small organ'. In cell biology the term refers to complex structures found only in eukaryotic cells, and not in prokaryotic cells, e.g. mitochondria, lisosomes, Golgi apparatus.

Penetrance   Penetrance refers to the extent to which a genetic variant has an effect on individuals who carry it. In practice it is the proportion of individuals that carry the mutated copy of the gene and express the phenotype (it is an indication of the 'strength' of the expression of the gene).

RNA   Ribonucleic acid. Single-stranded molecule formed by four different nitrogen bases (adenine (A), thymine (T), cytosine (C) and uracile (U)) that is found in all eukaryotic cells' cytoplasm and plays a vital role in transferring information from the DNA in the nucleus to the protein-forming apparatus in the cytoplasm (in which case it is called 'messenger RNA' or mRNA). (Increasingly, different types of RNAs have been identified with different roles; we only discuss mRNA in this volume.)

Single nucleotide polymorphism (SNP)   SNP refers to variations at the level of a single base pair in the DNA. These can be changes in a single base pair, deletions or insertions. SNPs may fall within coding sequences of genes, non-coding regions of genes, or in the intergenic regions between genes. Not always will SNPs within a coding sequence change the amino acid sequence of the protein that is produced, due to degeneracy (redundancy) of the genetic code. When DNA sequences from two homologous chromosomes contain a difference in a single nucleotide, we say they codify for two different alleles at a given genetic locus. If the variations affect more than one base pair they are called polymorphisms, not SNPs. In that case there is a higher chance that there will be some effect on the phenotype.

Somatic   Any cell that makes up an organism, except for gametes.

Zygote   A fertilised oocyte/egg is called a 'zygote'. It is produced by the fusion of two gametes.

INDEX

Note: italics indicate figures; 'n' indicates chapter notes.